Why and How We Get Sick:

Not by Witches and Wizards.

By

Rev. I.Felix A. Onyeise, MD, MS, CHHP, RDMS, NCAC11.

Table of Contents

Preface

This entire work is faith-based. Therefore, I preface it by emphasizing that our beliefs shape and determine our values, character, behavior, and actions. Our beliefs ultimately determine how we manage health. Contrary to the popular axiom to the effect that: seeing is believing, careful examination shows that what we believe influences what we see and what we hear. We also interpret what we see and hear in the context of what we believe.

Secondly, I would like to clarify an age-long misinformation by clergies of all denominations that puts human lifespan as three scores and ten years. This notion is a prayer of Moses found in the Holy Bible which I dub the **Manual of Life (MoL)**; Psalm 90:10 that states: "The days of our lives are seventy years; And if by reason of strength they are eighty years." (NKJV). However, our Creator gave us 120years. Genesis 6:3 states, "And the LORD said, 'My Spirit shall not strive with man forever, for he is indeed flesh; yet his days shall be one hundred and twenty years' (NKJV). That was how long Moses lived. Deuteronomy 34: 5-7 states, "So Moses the servant of the LORD died there in the land of Moab, according to the word of the LORD. And He buried him in a valley in the land of Moab, opposite Beth Peor; but no one knows his grave to this day. Moses was one hundred and twenty years old when he died. His eyes were not dim, nor his natural vigor diminished" (NKJV).

The implication of the three scores and ten misinformation is that its believers reach seventy years and unconsciously discard their survival instinct. Instead, they begin to live a reckless, I-don't-care lifestyle, on the assumption that additional years of life is a bonus. In one word, to reach the 120 years given by our Creator, depends on how we take care of our health which depends on what health information is available to us that we believe.

Health illiteracy is a challenge worldwide, much more so in Africa. In African countries, health illiteracy is the main cause of the high burden of diseases and premature deaths. Average life span in any African country is less than fifty years. This is compared to many western countries, where the average life span is above seventy-three years.

There are many factors responsible for the shortened life span in African countries. These factors include incompetent governance, poor hygiene, ill equipped healthcare facilities, under educated healthcare providers, lack of adequate continuing education for healthcare providers, adulterated and substandard drugs, misuse and abuse of drugs by self-prescription, superstitious beliefs, incompetent healthcare regulatory agencies, and paternalistic healthcare model. A complete book could be developed on each of these factors.

One umbrella that unites all these factors is health illiteracy, the hub, from which all these factors spin off. Therefore, educating Africans with evidence-based health information is one route to increased healthy lifespan. Acquiring and disseminating evidence-based health information rests on the shoulder of all Africans in a position to do so, many live in Africa and in the diaspora. Health illiteracy perpetuates beliefs in witches, wizards, superstition, (such as, generational curse and related myths) as cause of illness.

Medieval doctors (circa 476 AD to 1492 AD) in Western countries had no clue as to what caused diseases. Many doctors then believed in a humorism theory (perpetuated by Drs Hippocrates and Galen) which states that people became ill when “Four humors” namely, – phlegm, black bile, yellow bile, and blood are unbalanced. Subsequently, Dr Paracelsus proposed later that things that cause illness are from outside and not inside. During medieval period when people get sick and epidemic occur, these events were blamed on witches or scapegoats of different ethnicity (Jew) as cause. Other scapegoats include more or less inanimate objects like stars, demons, sin, and bad smell. Today, in the 21st century, many Africans still retain some of these medieval beliefs regarding the origins of diseases. This and other unscientific beliefs explain the impermissible low lifespan of Africans, in some countries less than 50 years, about the number circa 1842 in the West (52 years for the rich and 15 years for the poor) when the beliefs of causes of illness stood where many Africans stand today. These superstitious beliefs are reinforced in this 21st century by unscrupulous self-proclaimed African clergies, herbalists, prayer warriors, and even some conventional medical practitioners, who profit by deceiving the public to premature death.

Antibiotics were born In 1860 when Louis Pasteur discovered that germs (bacteria) caused infectious diseases. Following this discovery, Westerners embraced the new evidence-based truth and switched their beliefs. Scientists tapped into this new evidence in search of chemicals to kill the germs, leading to the birth of antibiotics. As a result, the health and lifespan of western countries began to rise and has maintained the rise with new evidence of true causes of illnesses and implementation of evidence-based treatment for them.

However, in Nigerian, and other African countries, beliefs in witches, wizards, voodoo, ghosts, and related evil spirits invoked by enemies within or outside the family still drives healthcare in the 21st century. Despite the fact that evidence-based health information is more abundant than ever, many African countries have not embraced evidence-based information for true cause of various illnesses. Elective ignorance and refusal to embrace evidence-based health facts by masses of Africans account for incomparable healthy lifespan with Western countries. There is a clear direct link between this tenacious hold on superstitious beliefs about causes of illness and the following: kidnapping, rituals, poverty, poor governance pervasive in Africa, and premature death. As the saying goes, it is what an individual believes and resources available to him, that ultimately determine the course of action that individual takes. Consequently, many sick Nigerians do not seek healthcare at all until it is too late, and when they lately do so, they go to prayer warriors, churches, herbalists, and native doctors, who milk them of what little money they have, before leaving them to their devices with consequences that range from permanent disability to premature death.

Besides poverty, the public has lost faith in the conventional healthcare system for various reasons. One such reason is how healthcare personnel treat patients. Be it private or government hospitals, and clinics, patients are dehumanized, and talked down to by the very same health personnel entrusted to relieve their pains and sufferings. More often than not, many patients who came with physical illness leave the hospital and clinic with permanent emotional and psychological scars. Such afflicted individuals seldom seek care from conventional health providers in the future.

To improve the health and life expectancy of Africans, the first and most important course of action is grass root public health education aimed at debunking these unfounded pristine mystical beliefs and related misinformation as causes of illness.

Introduction

We humans get sick because we are alive. The process of our early development is very complicated, and many mistakes do occur. The reality is, we must not only get sick as we live, but many of us are also born with sicknesses due to developmental errors. We get sick because we are living in a competitive world with various visible and invisible living things struggling to survive at the expense of one another. Recent scientific research strongly indicate that our body is home to about 30 trillion human cells and 39 trillion microbiomes (microorganisms), many of which are linked to our day-to-day normal body function while others can cause illnesses. The constant presence of microorganisms in us that can at any given time cause illness makes us potentially sick any minute. However, we do not become sick primarily due to our immune system's natural responsibility to keep these potentially disease-causing microorganisms in check. The moment the guard of the immune system is lowered to suboptimal, we become sick.

We also get sick because of what we eat and drink. Both quality, quantity and frequency of nutrient consumption are crucial. Some of us eat too much while others eat too little. We do not eat natural food today as our ancestors did. In our desperate and unguarded desire to emulate Westerners, we eat mostly processed food grown and treated with antibiotics and chemicals for fast growth, preservation, taste and looks. Many of the chemicals used in food production and processing are proven risks for many diseases. The food we eat today lack life-sustaining and health-promoting micronutrients (vitamins, minerals, and phytonutrients) due to depletion of nutrients of the soil on which they are planted. Deficiency of these micronutrients account for many illnesses we suffer. We equally get injured and become sick due to human errors, unsafe roads, misjudgment of risks and natural disasters.

Notice that there is no mention of witches and wizards as causes of any illnesses. This is because there is no concrete evidence available anywhere that witches and wizards exist, let alone causing any illness. Witches and wizards are constructs of the human mind. If you wish to know more about the reality of existence of witches and wizards, google for the history of witches and wizards on the internet. And it will prove to you that a human being produced the word witch and wizard with no such living entity in existence. We get sick because we are less physically active than before. Technology has provided facilitating machinery, for movement, farming and entertainment so we sit more and use less energy.

Another reason we get sick is due to ever increasing and persistent stress. Our personal lifestyle is a major cause of several illnesses. Various types of accidents, interpersonal conflicts, environmental and natural disasters are all sources of different illness. Despite reliable evidence showing otherwise, majority of Africans still believe that illnesses are caused by witches, wizards, evil spirits, and generation curse. And lastly but not the least in causing illness is misuse of drugs whether Western or native ones. Disease of drug addiction is at epidemic proportion in Nigeria and no witches, wizards or angry ancestors is making or importing the drugs.

The entrance door to knowledge and wisdom is wider today than ever, and many Africans do not have access to it primarily due to governmental corruption. In addition to what is written here, there are many authentic websites on the internet to learn evidence-based scientifically proven causes of illnesses, none of which lists witches, wizards, evil spirits, generational curse, and the like as cause.

This work is aimed primarily at educating African audiences about the true causes of illnesses, with the hope that many would come to know why and how we get sick, how not to get sick, and the right thing to do when at some point, we become sick. It would also enlighten non-Africans on why Africans have shorter life expectancy than their Western contemporaries. Knowledge is power. Armed with this right information, it is hoped that you, the reader, would then seek for healthcare at the right time, at the right place, and actively participate in your own healthcare, following medical advice to achieve best possible health, and improved lifespan.

Learn and live.

Chapter 1
Born Sick

Some of us are born sick and are said to have congenital sickness. Congenital means abnormal condition, such as deformity, illness, or disease that an individual was born with, which can initially appear as simple, non-symptomatic physical birth mark, or as multiple gross physical deformities. See **Figure 1.** Some birth marks may eventually develop into illness such as skin cancer at a later age. Many congenital problems are biochemical and not noticeable at birth until they manifest at a later age.

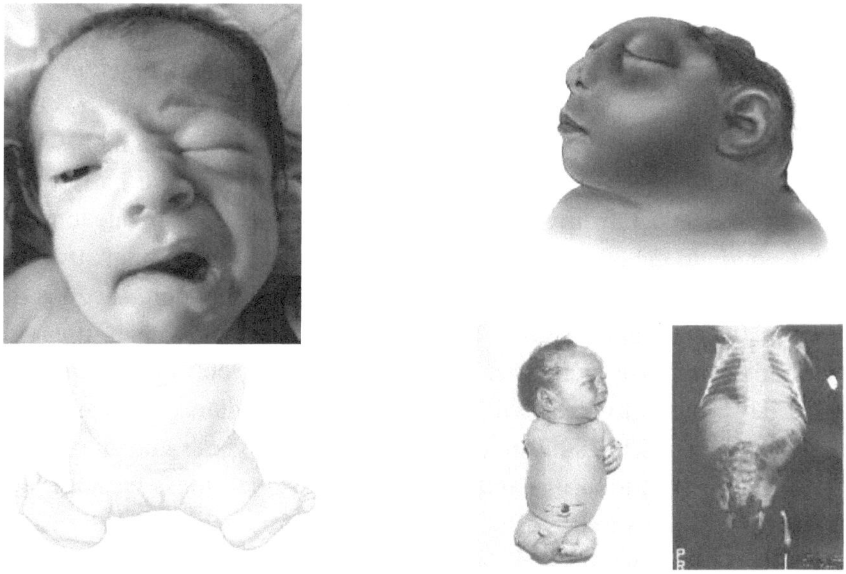

Figure 1

With time, some biochemical aberrations result in behavior, social or cognitive challenges with the affected individual unable to function normally in society. Some of these malformations are due strictly to nature's mistakes during early development in the uterus, or during evolutionary adaptation, while others are induced due to lifestyle of a pregnant mother, and the impregnating father. More on these later in the discussion on the role of lifestyle and environmental factors. Given the complexity of the processes involved in development of female egg (ovum), male sperm, process of ovulation, fertilization and growth that take place for the nine months of pregnancy before birth, nature's mistakes during early human development sometimes are inevitable. Those who studied embryology (study of early development) can easily appreciate the high potential for mistakes during early human development.

A little elementary biology here will help clarify things for us. For instance, our skin, teeth, nails, hair, muscles, and every part of our body may look very smooth to the naked eye. However, when any of these parts is placed under electron microscope, it becomes very clear that each human part is made of individual cells netted together cell-after-cell by connective tissue much the same way a block or brick wall is put together block-after-block with chunk of cement to hold them together. The connective tissue which functions like chuck of cement to hold individual cells together is composed of collagen and elastic fibers which are proteins. The connective tissue, which is a restrictive barrier that separates each cell from the other dictates what crosses from one location of the body to the other. A tissue is a group of cells with similar structure and work together to perform the same specialized function. A cell is the unit of structure and function of the human body, and as such, it is also the unit of disease or illness. When one cell or group of cells is sick, invariably the individual will be sick or ill. Cell damage during early development will result in congenital illness. The same applies to evolution. Evolutionary adaptation results in some illness because, just as an individual subjected to some harsh environments, like excessive cold or warmth, would seek a way to escape, so also is escape initiated at the cellular level when an unfavorable condition persists around cells. In such adverse conditions, cells will begin to rearrange their genetic code in an attempt to escape a persisting adverse condition. This adaptation by mutation may result in diseases. An example of one nucleotide replacement disease is sickle cell disease. In sickle cells, just one nucleotide, adenine, is replaced with thymine which resulted in valine amino acid replacing glutamic acid at the sixth position of beta globin of hemoglobin. This results in abnormal hemoglobin that elongates in absence or low oxygen tension leading to blood clotting and severe painful symptoms. F**igure 2** shows the difference in normal red blood cells and abnormal sickled cells of sickle cell disease, a result of adaptive mutation.

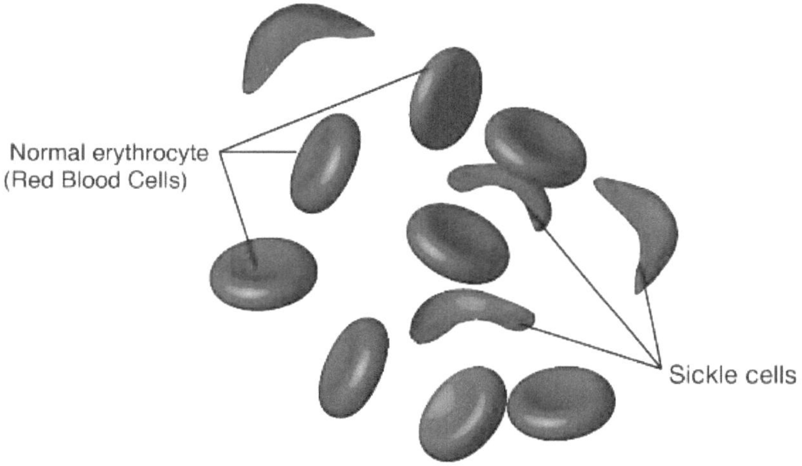

Figure 2

On a spate of good news, adaptation is not always negative. Instead, some adaptations result in positive conditions whereby the new product confers much better survival characteristics. A new area of study in cell biology is focusing on cell intelligence, asking questions like; how does a cell sense an adverse situation and seek to adjust to a more favorable structure? How does human immune deficiency virus (HIV) know to find a sanctuary within the same cell nature charged with destroying it.

Chapter 2
Diseases Resulting from Competition

One truth human beings ignore during their daily actions is the indisputable fact that we share this world with many other living things: some visible to the naked eye and many more not visible. This sharing of the same universe results in ever persisting competition for survival. The two primary goals of all living things are self-preservation through daily feeding and self-perpetuation through procreation. Both visible living things like humans, other animals, ants, and plants, as well as invisible living things like viruses, bacteria, worms, and fungi; all strive every second of the day to meet these two primary goals of self-preservation and perpetuation. For every organism to find food to eat and to beget and sustain their offspring are of most importance, and it is pursued at all costs, and unintentionally cause death of their neighbors, and destruction of their environment. It is therefore implicit that the most pressing challenge for all living things is to keep living. To keep living, a living thing must eat another living thing, and at the same time, protect itself from being eaten by another living thing. The food chain, **Figure 3** illustrates this disease and death-causing natural principle.

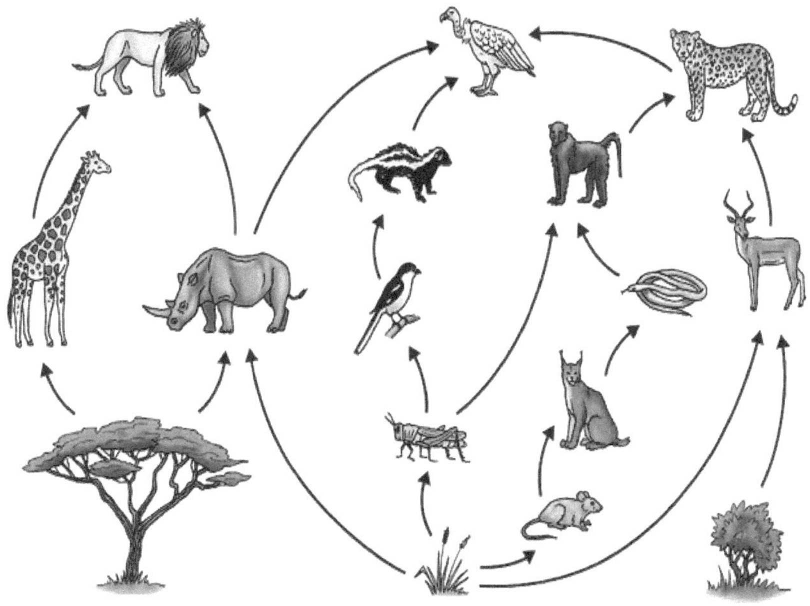

Figure 3

Members of the plant kingdom are the only living things that produce their own food by using energy from sunlight. Some living things eat only plants (like vegetables, fruits, nuts, and seeds), while others eat those that eat plants, while still others eat both plants and animals.

Invisible things like viruses, bacteria, worms, and fungi cannot produce their food, and cannot farm like humans to increase their food supply. They cannot survive independently. They must depend completely on other living things to obtain their food. Some viruses live in bacteria, worms, fungi, plants, and humans to sustain themselves. It is estimated that trillions of bacteria live within the human body. They are collectively known as microbiomes. Some make useful contributions to our health and are considered friendly, while others are potentially harmful when the conditions for such is right.

Obviously, when humans harvest vegetables, fruits, kill cow, goat, or fish for food, it results in the death of these edibles. To become food, the edible must die. However, the goal of the eater is not to destroy the edible, but rather to eliminate hunger, and obtain energy for strength to carry out life sustaining activities. Only plants through the energy from the sun can produce their own food without killing another living thing. It gets complicated when we realize that some water plants eat fish. When this table is turned against humans, by viruses, bacteria, worms, fungi, and ants, that obtain their food by living in or on humans, they cause damage that we refer to as sickness, specifically, infection. These parasites do not intend harm to their human host. In fact, they would prefer their host to remain perpetually alive so they will not run out of food. Unfortunately, the process of their obtaining food from their host if not halted will invariably lead to the death of the host. This is where the immune system comes in, to protect the host from being destroyed by a parasite that only wants food but is naïve of the reality that the process is causing damage that could lead to the death of its host and ultimately to its own death. **Figure 4** illustrates some infections caused by parasites.

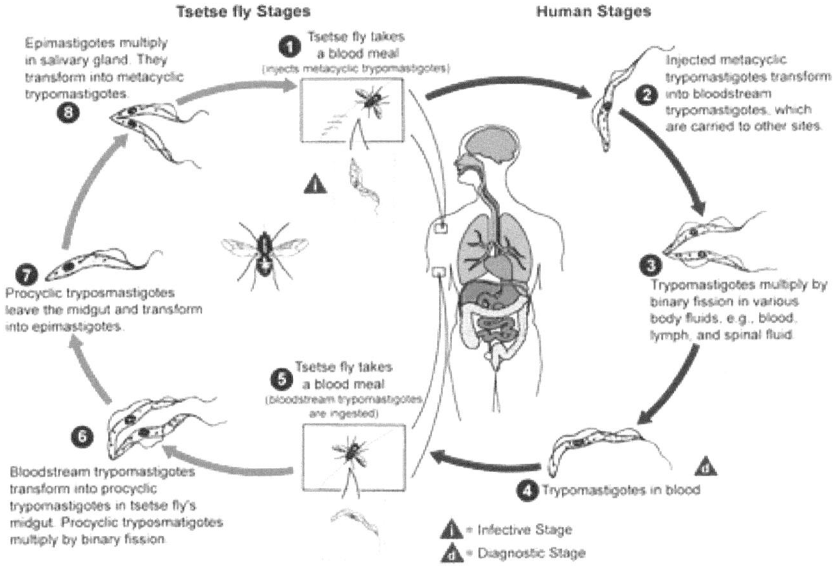

Figure 4

Note that not all association with these microorganisms is detrimental to humans. Emerging research shows that lots of the bacteria inside the human body play a life sustaining role, including enhancing the immune system and brain function.

Chapter 3
Micronutrient Deficiency Diseases.

One reality all humans ought to accept but may not cherish is the fact that all living things, both visible and invisible, plants and animals alike, will at one time or the other, or even many times in the life cycle get sick. Contemporary Nigerians deny this unavoidable fact by hiding behind, "I reject it, it is not my portion, Holy Ghost fire." But the Holy Ghost carries neither matches nor cigarette lighters. "I do not claim it," and a neighbor echoes the same, "sister do not claim it." Either you claim it and do something about it, or it will claim you. These misguided Nigerians are being deceived by their so-called spiritual guides and clergy. However, the reality of disease in living things is so true that the Creator and Author of life in anticipation of this very truth, equipped all living things with a defense system to protect them from potential sickness-causing agents and events. In the case of humans, the protective defense system is known as the immune system. This system is perhaps the next most sophisticated human system after the nervous system which includes the brain. The immune system is composed of diverse specialized cells that perform their individual nature assigned duty diligently. These cells work collectively and cooperatively to achieve a common goal of recognizing and destroying any foreign invader of the body, such as (viruses, bacteria, worms, and fungi) or normal self-cell that becomes abnormal (cancer), and aged nonfunctional cell. These immune cells manufacture their own bullets and bombs, (weapons of mass destruction, so to say), in the form of chemicals collectively known as cytokines. Some families of cytokines are interleukins, interferons, mesenchymal growth factors, chemokines, tumor necrosis factors, and adipokines.

Each human is unique, and the immune cells know this natural fact better than anything else. The core function of the immune system is to offer protection to the human body. It is naturally programmed to recognize cell surface proteins, which distinguish non-self-cells, (invaders) and altered normal self-cells, such as (cancer cells, aged and dead cells) from normal self-cells. All the normal cells of an individual's body are recognized as self and are free of attack. However, when a self-cell becomes cancerous or aged and nonfunctional, the surface protein changes, and it is recognized as foreign and destroyed. All invaders of the body are also recognized as enemies because their surface protein is different from that of the normal self-cell; consequently, the enemy is destroyed. **Figure 5** depicts the complexity and sophistication of the immune cells in action.

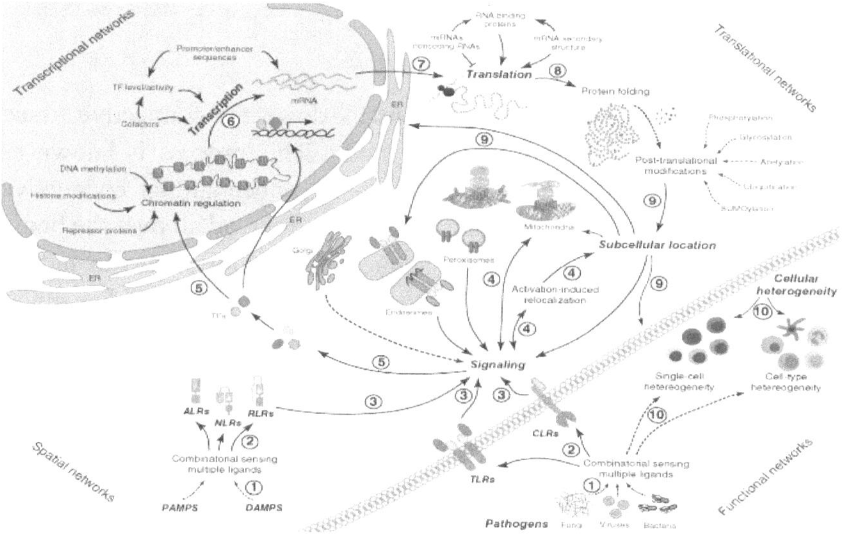

Figure 5

The immune cells deploy cytokines in two different ways to perform their function. Some cytokins directly kill invaders or altered cells while others activate and summon more cells to the location of the invader or altered cell. Immune cells use cytokines to rid the body of damaged and aged nonfunctioning cells. Some cytokines do the actual killing and others function like the cellphone (call 911) to recruit more cells to the location of killing attack. It gets even more complex when it is recognized that both the invader and altered self-cells that are being attacked stage counter defense attack, using their own produced chemicals. Normally, the connective tissue links cells together and at the same time functions as a barrier restricting movement from one location of the body to the other. See **Figure 6**.

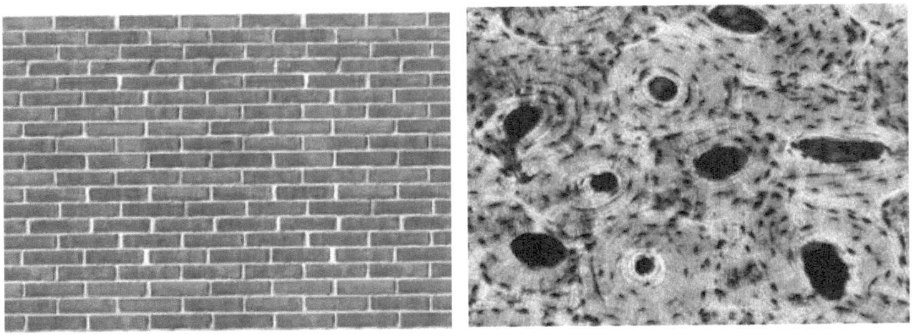

Figure 6

Cancer cells produce chemicals that break down the connective tissue allowing them to spread all over the body. This process is known as cancer metastasis. Some parasitic invaders produce similar connective tissue destructive molecules that enable them to spread all over the body. Cancer cells also produce other chemicals that allow them to induce formation of new blood vessels (angiogenesis) through which they divert nutrients and oxygen away from normal cells for their selfish rapid growth. Immune cells fight back against these cancer cell-disease processes by producing various specific cytokines that tend to inhibit both metastasis and angiogenesis. Success by the immune system requires it to be maintained in optimally competent state accomplished only by steady supply of adequate amount of macro and micronutrients. When optimal nutrients are supplied, the immune system will conquer cancer and related illnesses and produce a cure. When the immune system is incompetent due to lack of or inadequate supply of one or more macro or micronutrient, cancer and other illnesses progress and lead to death. Unaware to humans, is the constant ongoing biological and chemical warfare inside our body. We survive each day because a competent immune system wins these wars most of the time. One way we get sick is when the immune system is incompetent or not functioning at its optimal capacity due to deficiency of one or more macro and/or micronutrients.

To manufacture molecular weapons of mass destruction known as cytokines, the immune cells require raw materials; in the form of macronutrients (carbohydrates, protein, and fat) and micronutrients, (vitamins, minerals, and phytochemicals) all of which are found in balanced nutrition or as commercially available supplements. In the absence of these essential critical nutrients, the immune cells will not be able to face off against invaders and cancer cells. So, when malnutrition exists, the immune system will fail, and invaders and cancer cells will have the upper hands to sustain illness. The biology behind cancer development is not completely understood. What we do know is that certain environmental factors and even some drugs and radiation used to treat cancer are known to cause cancer by altering the genetic code. There is also theoretical speculation that deficiency of one or more micronutrients critical as a co-enzyme in genetic building, modification, and repair may result in malfunction of gene coding, leading to cancer development.

During early childhood, especially the first six months of life, the immune system is not quite developed, and the infant is primarily dependent on antibodies (proteins produced and used by immune cells to fight diseases) in the breast milk to fend off disease-causing invaders.

As humans get older, the immune system's ability to manufacture cytokines decreases for various reasons, such as poor nutrition, decreased efficiency of biochemical reactions, and enzyme deficiency, due partly to lack of co-enzymes (micronutrients). Micronutrients, such as vitamins and minerals, act as co-enzymes in many biochemical reactions responsible for manufacturing cytokines. A combination of poor nutrition and inability of the aging human body to extract enough vitamins, minerals, and phytochemicals from food handicaps the immune system and results in micronutrient deficiency diseases. **Table 1** lists some known disease symptoms caused by micronutrient deficiency.

NUTRITIONAL DEFICIENCIES

Experiencing these symptoms? Some of these nutrients might help!

EMOTIONAL		**MOUTH**	
Fatigue	Iron	Cracked lips	Vitamin B12
Anxiety	B Complex	Weak teeth	Vitamin D, Calcium
Depression	Vitamin D	Sore tongue	B Complex
Poor memory	Vitamin D, B complex	Bleeding gums	Vitamin C, Folate
HAIR		**NAILS**	
Dandruff	Omega 3, Selenium	Brittleness	Calcium, Magnesium
Breakage	Biotin Omega 3, Vitamin E	Paleness	Biotin, Iron
Thinning	Biotin, Vitamin D, Zinc	White spots	Calcium, Zinc
SKIN		**MUSCLES**	
Dryness	Omega 3, Vitamin A & E	Cramping	Magnesium, Potassium
Bruising	Iron, Vitamin C	Numbness	B Complex
Inflammation	B Complex, Biotin	Twitching	B Complex, Calcium, Magnesium, Vitamin D
EYES		**JOINTS**	
Dark circles	Iron	Clicking	Manganese, Omega 3
Poor vision	Vitamin A & D	Swelling	B Complex Potassium

Table 1.

The human body continues to develop and reach growth peak at about age twenty-five to thirty. During the growth period, the efficiency of the biochemical processes is at its optimal state. Extraction of micronutrients from food is optimal. However, after the peak age of twenty-five to thirty, all the biochemical processes of the human body begin to decline gradually **Figure. 7.** Henceforth, the body requires supplementation of micronutrients to enable efficient biochemical reactions for the immune system to continue its all-important protection. Even before age twenty-five, depending on availability of foods and types of food available to an individual, hereditary deficiencies, and diseases the individual already has, supplementation with micronutrients may be needed to augment what is available from food. Deficiency of one or more micronutrients will also result in disease during this critical growth period. For example, rickets was ravaging children worldwide until 1920 when Vitamin D deficiency was discovered as the cause of the illness. Currently, vitamin D deficiency has been implicated in various diseases. Current knowledge indicates that Vitamin D is not actually a vitamin, because the human body can produce it from sunshine. A vitamin is an essential factor for life that the human body does not produce. Vitamin D is now said to be a prohormone (substance used as a basic molecule to produce many other substances). Optimal Vitamin D level in human body is now considered so critical to good health that it must be maintained to avoid various diseases. Some scientists have dubbed it "molecule of life." Thus, medical scientists have designated November second of each year as Vitamin D Day. For more information on Vitamin D and various diseases its deficiency has been linked to visit www.vitamindcouncil.org.

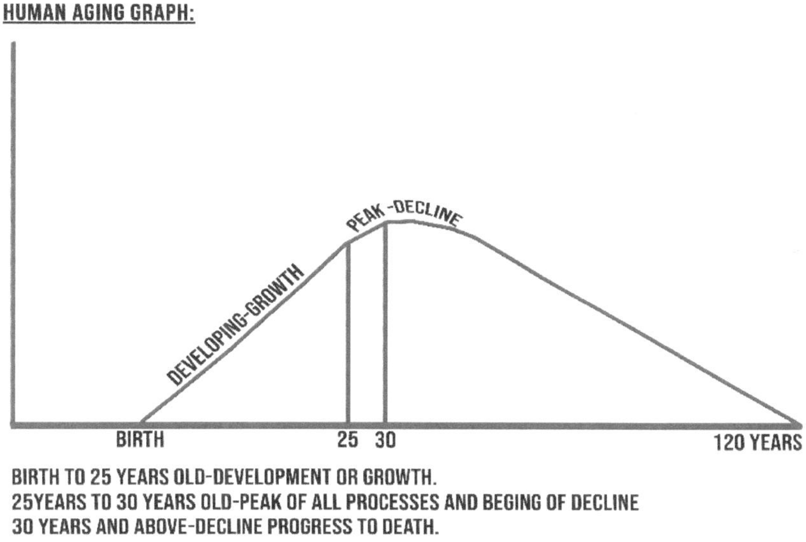

Fig. 7

Dr. Mathias Rath is a pioneer natural healthcare research scientist living in California who has built upon earlier discovery of Vitamin C deficiency as the cause of a devastating disease known as scurvy, which was said to have killed over two million sailors during the age of sailing. Dr Rath has shown that chronic deficiency of Vitamin C contributes to the cause and sustaining of many chronic diseases, such as (heart diseases, high blood pressure, diabetes, and high cholesterol), that plague the world, and account for numerous premature deaths worldwide. He has demonstrated the role of micronutrients' deficiencies in causing diseases, and how adequate supplementation with the deficient micronutrient could restore healing and cure disease. His findings are published in his seminal, **Why Animals don't Heart Attacks-But**

People Do! Fourth Revised Edition (Fremont, CA: MR Publishing, Inc. 2003).

It is clear that when the body cells lack wholly or partially the natural micronutrients, essential or nonessential amino acids, which are crucial for them to carry out their naturally programmed functions, they malfunction and disease results. Consequently, one can infer that numerous diseases begin at the level of the basic unit of life: the cell. Thus, the resulting disease type depends on what micronutrient is deficient and which cells are affected. A deficiency suffered by B-cells of the pancreas which normally produce insulin will result in B-cells inability to produce insulin needed for glucose absorption. Complete lack of insulin will result in diabetic disease while reduced insulin production may result in glucose intolerance. Vitamin D has been shown to play a significant role in insulin production and secretion, and its deficiency is implicated as a contributing factor in the cause of Type-Two diabetes.

Chapter 4
Immune Deficiency and Autoimmune Diseases

The immune system can also overreact and result in other types of diseases. Medical science does not know completely why the immune system, naturally designed to protect the body, sometimes overreact to cause diseases such as allergies. Inflammation is one hallmark of the immune system process to combat diseases. Normally inflammation should cease once a disease condition is averted. However, this is not always the case. Sometimes inflammation persists and becomes a disease of its own. It is believed that almost all chronic diseases have inflammatory components. Many biochemical reactions have a built-in feedback control system that limits the forward reaction. For example, in the production of estrogen hormone, when the amount required to carry out normal physiologic function is produced, estrogen will shut down the enzyme that controls its production. If this feedback control fails, production of estrogen will be sustained infinitely, resulting in a level that would be toxic to the point of becoming a disease. In that case, the control mechanism for inflammation fails, and it becomes sustained as chronic inflammation, a disease of its own. Another process by which the immune system causes diseases is mistaken identity. In this case a normal cell is mistaken as an invader, and gets destroyed, because an invader has a surface-recognition protein very close in structure to that of a normal cell. These types of diseases are known as autoimmune diseases. **Table 2** lists examples of autoimmune diseases.

Accepted Autoimmune Diseases

- Addison's Disease
- Autoimmune Inner Ear Disease (AIED)
- Balo Disease
- Behcet's Disease
- Bullous Pemphigoid
- Chronic Fatigue Immune Dysfunction Syndrome (CFIDS)
- Chronic Inflammatory Demyelinating Polyneuropathy
- Cicatrical Pemphigoid
- Cold Agglutinin Disease
- CREST Syndrome
- Crohns Disease
- Dermatomyositis
- Diabetes Mellitus Type 1
- Goodpasture's Syndrome
- Graves' Disease
- Guillain-Barre Syndrome (GBS)
- Hashimoto's Disease
- Juvenile Arthritis
- Lichen Planus
- Lupus Erythematosus
- Meniere's Disease
- Myasthenia Gravis Narcolepsy
- PANDAS
- Pemphigus Vulgaris
- Pernicious Anemia
- Psoriatic Arthritis
- Polymyositis
- Primary Biliary Cirrhosis
- Rheumatoid Arthritis
- Sjogren's Syndrome
- Ulcerative Colitis
- Vasculitis
- Wegener's Granulomatosi

Coronado Biosciences

19

Table 2.

Chapter 5
Stress-Related Disease

What is stress? Is it bad, all the time? Or is there something good about it? What is the difference between stress and distress? Stress is a response by the human body to any kind of demand which can be emotional, psychological, spiritual, or physical. Stress is a natural response meant to spur one into action. Stress response is supposed to be protective. It somehow motivates you into action. When a student is facing an examination, it provokes stress, and he responds by studying hard. Stress is an involuntary response to a sense of danger, whether real or imagined. A stressor is anything real or imagined that leads to stress response. The body's response to stress is not voluntary. It involves involuntary release of hormones and neurotransmitters, such as (epinephrine, norepinephrine, and cortisol) which prepares the individual to either stay and fight or flee the danger. This is known as a fight or flight response. Anyone interested in the details of this important physiological response can Google it. Acute stress that elicits acute stress-response may not be damaging to the body as the released hormones and neurotransmitters do metabolize quickly and the response stops. However, when a stressor persists, the stress response also persists with the neurotransmitters and hormones released remaining ever present and result in either body damage or behavior that is out of norm for society. At this point, stress metamorphoses into distress, capable of causing sickness. Chronic persisting stress response has been shown to cause heart diseases and as major risk for various cancers especially breast cancer. If someone suddenly runs into a snake, his heart will immediately begin beating faster and more intense, muscles become tightened with increased blood flow into them in preparation to get the person out of danger. The snake may also run away in response to seeing human as a stressor. Once escape from danger is achieved, in this case the snake, production of stress hormones and neurotransmitters ceases and reabsorption of neurotransmitters and hormones produced occur. The person's muscles relax, and rapid heartbeat and breathing will calm down to normal. But what if the stressor is mythical belief in make-believe phenomena like witches, wizards, and evil spirit? There is as yet no scientific evidence supporting the existence of witches, wizards, and evil spirits. If an individual maintains in his or her imagination, images of these unreal phenomena, he or she will perpetually live with anxiety, depression, sleepless nights, and psychological pain. In this case, the stressor, a false belief tormenting the mind, perpetually and chronically sustains the stress response.

The lesson in all this is that reducing stress or managing stress is an important way to prevent several illnesses. One important common, and effective way to manage stress is prayer. Those who have physical illness benefit from decreased stress hormones that calms them down, but the physical illness requires additional specific treatment to heal. In the Bible, introduced before in this book as the Manual of Life, MoL, the Author of Life admonished that His creature should not be anxious about anything and instead must pray all the time (Philippians 4:6 NIV). Exercise is anti-stress. Walking for thirty minutes daily is enough to cause the body to release soothing natural relaxation, pain reducing hormones and neurotransmitters; endorphins, enkephalins, serotonin and dopamine. Vigorous exercise is not required as it can become a stressor to the body.

Meditation, yoga, tai chi, tai gong, massage and several other Chinese, African and Indian alternative treatments like acupuncture are stress-reduction techniques to be discussed shortly in this book.

Chapter 6
Personal Lifestyle-Related Diseases

Lifestyle denotes the way we live, including what we eat and drink, how often and how much we eat, daily sedentary and physical activities, hobbies, recreational activities, occupation, living environment, personal hygiene, religious activities, and social involvement. Each of these engagements can influence the state of our health in several ways. For instance, what a pregnant woman does affects herself and her unborn child. A pregnant woman eats and drinks for herself and her unborn child. What she eats or drinks that may not harm her, can be detrimental to the unborn child. A classical common example is a congenital group of damages known as fetal alcohol spectrum disorder; a result of drinking while pregnant. See **Figure 8.**

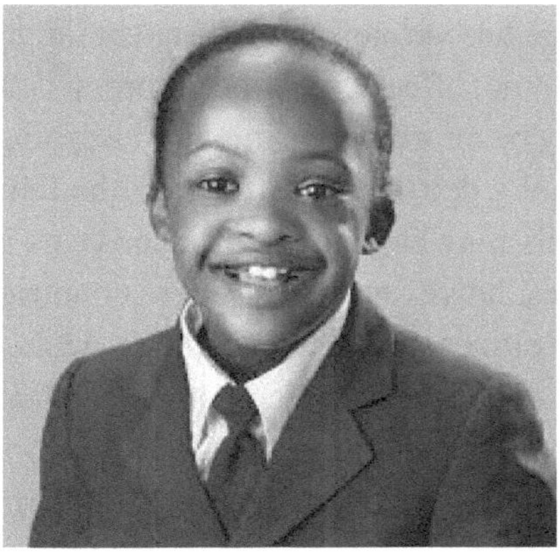

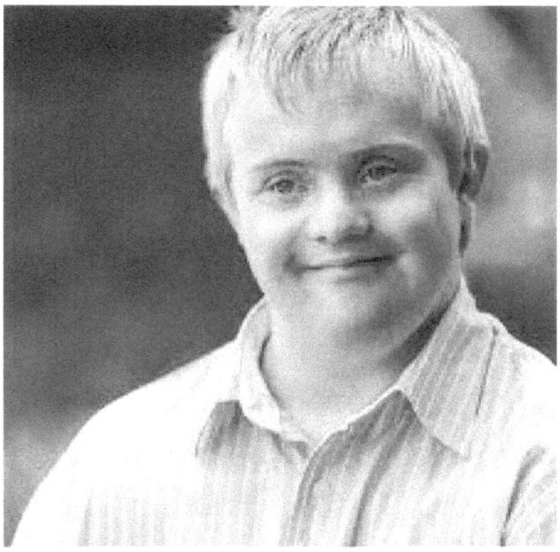

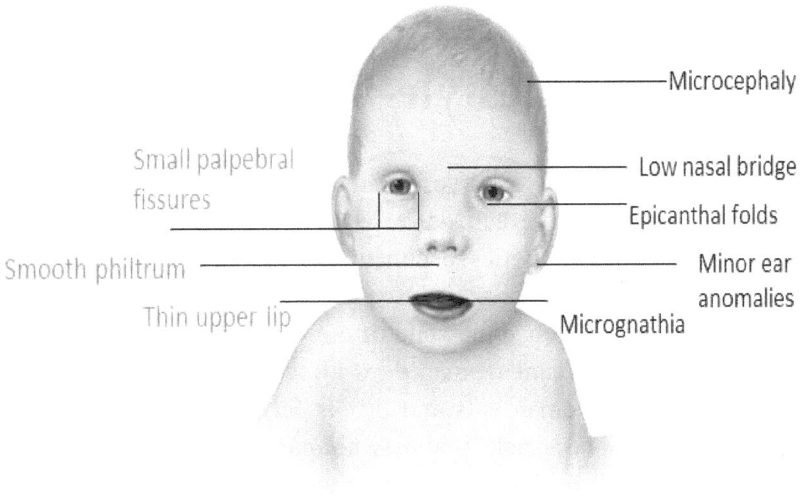

Figures 8

Spectrum means that the manifestation has variable gradation that ranges from mild to severe expression. Some effects may be expressed as physical appearance while others may be expressed as impaired learning, or social and behavior ability. Alcohol's detrimental effects on the fetus may be seen early at birth while others may be delayed till later years in life. Alcohol is legal in many countries; however, only Western countries specify the legal ages at which their citizens can start drinking alcohol. The minimum age in many Western countries at which people can start drinking is 18 years old. In the USA, not too long ago, it was raised to 21 years. To the best of my knowledge, no African country has age limit at which their citizen should start drinking. However, Muslims in various African countries are expected not to drink at all in accordance with the Quran. That excessive alcohol consumption for a prolonged time has adverse effects to all organs of the human body is undisputed among research scientists. What is not clear yet is the quantity, how often and for how long alcohol is to be consumed before it results in illnesses. There is evidence-based fact that neither a woman about to get pregnant or already pregnant should drink alcohol of any type in any quantity at any time. Thus, in Western countries, alcohol bottles have what is known as black box warning in bold highlighted letters that reads; thus;

Government warning (1) According to the surgeon general, women should not drink alcohol beverages during pregnancy because of the risk of birth defects. (2) Consumption of alcohol beverages impairs your ability to drive a car or operate machinery and may cause health problems. In other words, scientist have agreed on zero tolerance of alcohol by pregnant women or women trying to get pregnant. Some people have questioned why alcohol, which for so long has been glamorously tolerated as a social lubricant, would have such strict restrictions for would-be or expectant mothers.

The answer to this question is that fetal alcohol spectrum disorder is real and results in children who remain challenged for the rest of their lives. The medical, social, and economic costs of raising such affected children through their lifespan to the family and society is staggering. The evidence of adverse effects of excess alcohol consumption by potential fathers to an unborn child is less obvious. However, it is known that heavy alcohol consumption over time alters the hormone balance in men which may result in less sperm production and ultimately in male infertility. Excessive prolonged alcohol consumption has been linked to cancer of all human organs, inflammation of the pancreas (pancreatitis), liver (fatty liver, hepatitis, cirrhosis, and liver cancer), inflammation of the entire gastrointestinal system (mouth, esophagus, stomach, small intestine, large intestine, and rectum), thinning of bone (osteoporosis), hypertension, seizures, malnutrition, and memory loss. No other drug, (yes, alcohol is a drug) affects the entire human body system more adversely than excessive prolonged imbibement of any type of alcohol.

Alcohol has unimpeded access to all cells of the human body because it is fat soluble and cell membranes are loaded with fat. Unlike other drugs, alcohol does not need special membrane surface protein (receptor) to assist it to enter cells. A more detailed discussion on the adverse effects of alcohol on human life will be available in a future booklet titled: **Alcohol A Drug that Kills.**

Best available research-evidence prohibits all smokables, whether: cigarette, tobacco, marijuana, or the like, for pregnant women and all humans. Nonetheless, the first two are universally legal while marijuana is legal in some countries. In Western countries, all smokable products are packaged with a written black box warning notice on the package to the effect that **smoking clogs arteries and can lead to heart attack and strokes.** Smoking by a pregnant woman causes premature labor and delivery of premature underweight baby. If such babies survive, they tend to encounter lifelong health challenges. The adverse effects to unborn babies caused by cigarette and tobacco apply to both active smoking (pregnant woman smoking) and passive smoking (pregnant woman inhaling smoke from someone smoking). Research studies show that children whose parents smoke develop asthma more often than those children whose parents do not smoke. Similarly, people living with smokers tend to develop lung cancer more often than those living with non-smokers. Smoke here applies to all smokable products. Marijuana (in Nigeria called **guuf,** as in **go-off**) is a risk for schizophrenia (craziness) in a predisposed individual, especially in teenagers. We all have witnessed the devastating effect of **(Mpkuru miri),** concocted mixture of various street drugs, many unidentified, but usually includes marijuana. Marijuana has been linked to infertility in men who smoke it chronically. It is also linked to chromosome damages that may result in birth to intellectually challenged children. In recent years, marijuana is being touted as medicinal, but the story is very complicated and there is no actual scientific research documentation of measurable results to support these philosophical medicinal effect claims. However, the jury is still out, given that there is ongoing research investigating these claims. So far, there is credible evidence that a derivative molecule from marijuana, known as Cannabidiol **(CBD)** oil, which is not addictive, reduce the frequency of seizures in epileptic patients. Until results from more rigorous-conducted research confirm authenticity of medicinal claims of marijuana, smoking it is not recommended by this author. More research evidence abound regarding its adverse, than positive effects.

Due to ethical reasons, many prescription drugs have not been evaluated for effects on unborn child. As a result, they are prohibited for use by pregnant women. Some prescription drugs are known to have adverse effects on unborn children and are strictly prohibited for use by pregnant women. USA Federal Drug Agency (equivalent of drug Control, NAFDAC, in Nigeria) has a lettered classification of all prescription drugs. Prescription drugs listed under letter C, are drugs on which not enough research has been conducted to determine if they are safe for use by pregnant women. The drugs under letter D, denote products that are harmful to unborn fetus and should, therefore, not be used by pregnant women. Sadly, the same drugs prohibited in pregnancy, and every other drug, are littered for free access in chemists and pharmacies all over Nigeria, to be purchased by anyone at any time. A clear example is the case of a drug known as thalidomide given to pregnant women all over Europe and USA years ago. See **Figures 9** for its devastating effect before it was pulled off market.

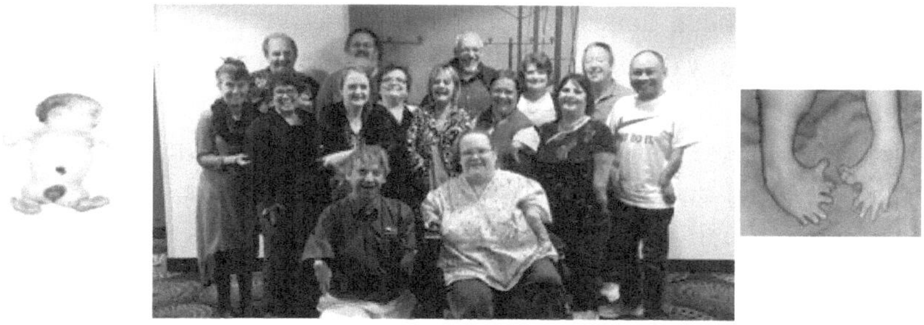

Figure 9

Children born of pregnant women who took thalidomide had devastating malformation with lack of limbs formation as most prominent.

Personal diet is most important in achieving and maintaining good health. No dispute, excessive consumption of table sugar, carbohydrates and products made from flour is a confirmed risk for various chronic debilitating illnesses like diabetes, high blood pressure, high cholesterol, cancers, and arthritis. Sugars, carbohydrates, and flour products provide mainly energy and lack much of the micronutrients relevant for the work of the immune system in defending the body from developing and healing illness. Excluding vegetables, fruits, and nuts (sources of micronutrients) from diet deprives the individual the phytonutrients (phytochemicals) necessary to optimize the protective role of the immune system. Lack of exercise is also a documented risk for chronic disease. Working long hours, without adequate resting period in-between, and sleep deprivation are all risk for various illnesses.

Chapter 7
Accident-Related Diseases.

We get sick from numerous types of accidents, including falls from bicycling, climbing, walking, driving, airplane, and industrial machinery mishaps. Human error and poor judgement can lead to various accidents that result in sickness. An unfavorable environment can precipitate accidents. A slippery wet floor can lead to a fall when care is ignored resulting in broken bones. Alcohol and addictive drugs lead to various accidents while walking, climbing, or driving. One example is case of a drunk driver, who is experiencing impaired judgement, and driving on one of countless single lanes, filled with potholes, which go-for roads in Nigeria. Head-on collision with oncoming vehicle from opposite direction is usually inevitable on these death-trap roads. See **Figure 10**.

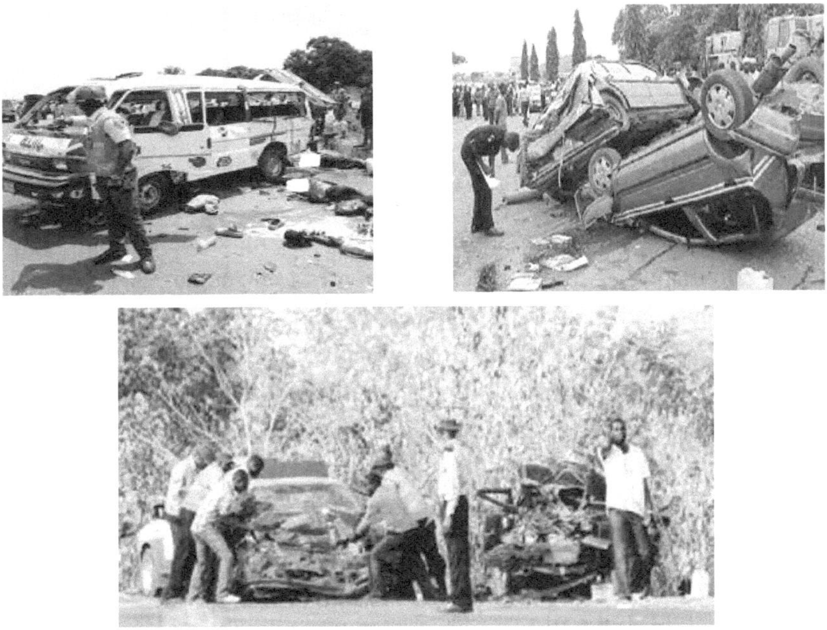

Figures 10.

Usually when accidents occur on these roads with or without an intoxicated driver involved, people will produce various versions of stories as to how the driver or someone in either of the vehicles has been bewitched to cause the accident. But the true witches and wizards responsible for the accident are four folds: the negligent governance model of government that ignores the bad road, road safety regulatory board agents who take bribe and ignore implementing safety rules, a poorly maintained vehicle, and the intoxicated or sleepy driver. Thus, combination of narrow multiple pot-holed roads and drunk driving results in thousands of deaths and permanent disability annually that is blamed on the machination of evil spirits. You may like to visit orthopedic hospital Enugu for hard evidence. Alcohol and drug intoxication lead to interpersonal fights resulting in injury and sometimes death. But illnesses resulting from these human accidents and dysfunctional lifestyle of drug addiction, and excessive alcohol consumption are ignorantly attributed to generational curses and witchcraft.

Natural disasters cause not only destruction of properties, injuries, and death at the time they occur, they also alter the environment such as flooding of rivers and sewage, which results in exploding growth of bacteria and other parasites leading to endemic diseases. Africans are lucky when it comes to natural disasters; many parts of the continent are devoid of hurricanes, tsunami, deadly volcanic eruption, mud slide, fire, and tornado. See **Figure 11** none of each took place in Africa.

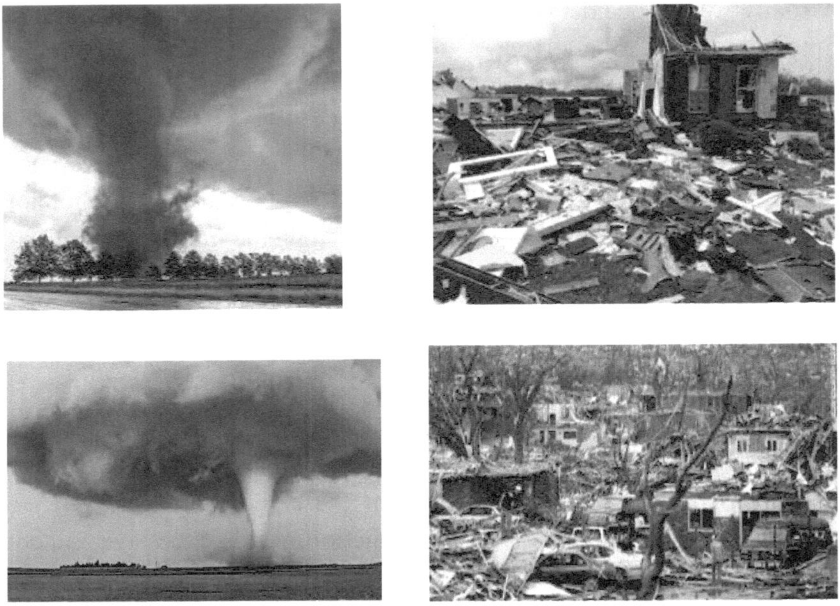

Figure 11

Flooding occurs in Nigeria and other African countries due to government negligence of erosion control. However, when there is a natural disaster, it is quickly said to have resulted from either punishment from God or due to attack by evil spirits. Diseases that follow natural events are equally ascribed to act of evil spirits, witchcraft, and punishment of ancestral curse. Outbreaks of cholera from contamination of drinking water after flood result in large number of deaths. Open sewage and gutters, accumulate a soup of stagnant water that allows for fermentation of rotting trash to release germs in the air that are inhaled by humans, resulting in serious fatal illnesses. **Figure 12**

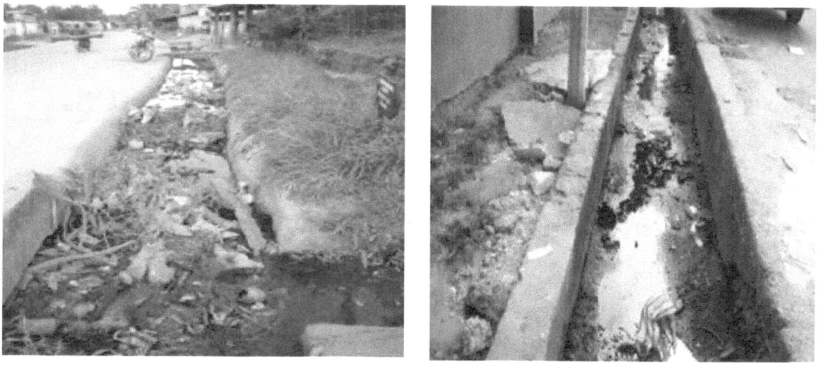

Figure 12

Similarly, these man-created occurrences are attributed to witches and wizards. In contrast, Western nations know that open gutters are sources of deadly illness, hence all gutters they built are completely covered.

Chapter 8
Environment Related diseases.

Some sickness results from how we manage our environment. As illustrated earlier, we are in competition with countless co-occupants of the environment. In their quest for survival, bacteria and other parasites colonize both the inside and outside of our bodies. Taking a bath at least once a day is a necessity to decrease the number of parasites on our body. Not taking a bath a significant number of days will result in overgrowth of these parasites and lead to infection. Ring worm and athletic foot caused by fungi are familiar examples. Why not blame these ones too on evil spirits? Regular adequate personal hygiene and a clean environment will preclude or mitigate certain sicknesses. Malaria responsible for the premature deaths of countless persons in sub-Sahara Africa, especially children and pregnant women are preventable if our environment are kept free of stagnant water. More on malaria prevention in the next section.

We are all familiar with flooding rivers, ponds, gutters, and potholes, during the rainy season. We are also equally familiar that if no one is looking, people urinate and defecate in the bushes and wherever else they fancy, including bushes surrounding market squares. Then comes flooding which carries all the wastes defecated in the bushes back to village and city markets. Now picture a market you have been to, like Nkwo Mbaise, Orie Mbaise, Eke Nguru, Afor Ogbe, Eke Oha Owerri, Port Harcourt, Abuja, Lagos markets, you can recall that crayfish, vegetables, fish, melon seed, pumpkin seed and much more edibles are displayed on a mart on ground level. See **Fig 13.**

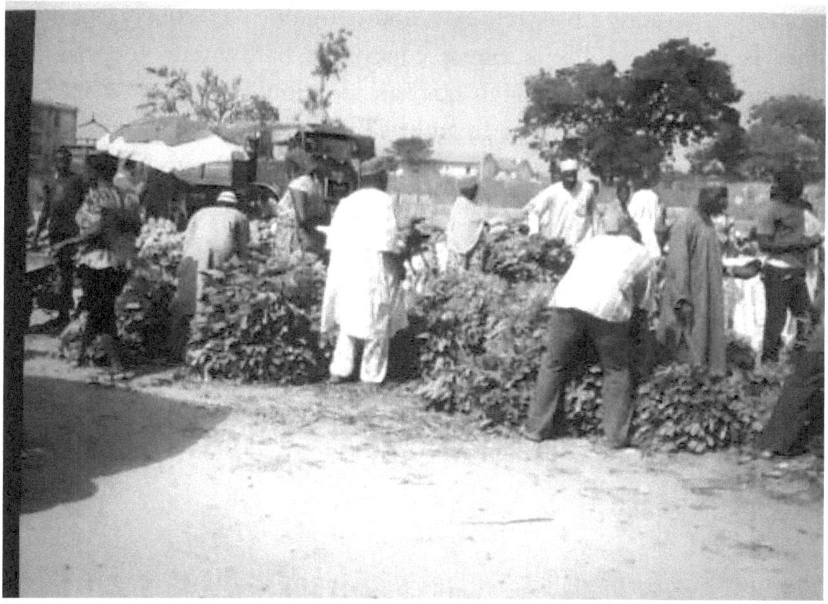

Figure 13

As buyers walk around shopping, they shove sand and dust contaminated by spores and eggs of parasites brought back by floods onto the displayed edibles.

Convincing scientific evidence shows that many parasitic eggs can survive temperatures above a hundred degrees, as well as survive hundreds of years in the environment, and still germinate when the condition is favorable. A very good example is ascaris worm (round worm) egg, a common parasitic infection in children of sub-Saharan Africa. Eggs of ascaris found in Egyptian mummy after over two thousand years still germinated in a favorable condition. Eggs of this worm and other worms have been heated in over one hundred degrees temperature and they still survived. It follows that if crayfish or vegetable contaminated by ascaris eggs from the market is not washed off properly, an unwashed off ascaris egg is likely to survive when it gets into the intestine of a human. Still some environmental factors, such as airborne dust, mold, animal dander, grass and plant pollens that cause asthma, allergies and hay fever are not easily amenable to human control. It is quite reasonable to ask why, of two friends sitting in the park, one person has a runny nose, red eyes and coughing vigorously, while the other is just fine. This is where genes; the hardwired blueprint, that humans are born with, which confers individual uniqueness interacts with environmental factors to unleash reactions from a predisposed individual and leaves the unpredisposed individual untouched. It does not mean that the man with running nose and coughing has seen a ghost, bewitched or victim of generational curse. His immune system is uniquely reacting to environmental factors in the air, and this happens to predisposed individuals worldwide. It is never due to witches, wizards, and evil spirits.

Chapter 9
How Not to Get Sick

The first section uncovers various things and ways available scientific evidence has shown through which we get sick. We get sick due to errors in complex processes involved during our formation in the womb, deficiency in the cell of natural building ingredients and enzymes God imbedded in plants and fruits as vitamins, minerals, and phytochemicals essential to maintain and sustain our health, competition for survival by all living things within the same environment, and unhealthy lifestyle. Other sources of getting sick include eating unhealthy food, eating too much or too little of healthy food, drinking alcohol excessively, smoking, natural disasters, accidents, and man-made alteration of the environment with pollution and production of harmful chemicals. There is no evidence that witches, wizards, ghosts, or evil spirits (if they exist) play any roles in causing any of the sicknesses. The human mind is powerful, and what you put into it becomes what it uses to direct your actions and behavior. We must then be mindful of what we believe. Belief in witches, wizards, evil spirits, and ghosts when internalized into the depths of our mind entirely control our behaviors and actions. These age-long superstitious beliefs induce and sustain fear in the mind. And this deep-seated fear-factor takes over our healthcare behavior.

When symptoms like fever, headache, stomachache, dizziness, vomiting, diarrhea appear, we head straight to native doctors or prayer warriors because we believe that these symptoms are due to attacks by evil spirits, witches and wizards sent by enemies. We do not go to conventional doctors and hospitals because they do not deal with what we believe is the cause of our symptoms.

Therefore, the most important step in adopting measures of how not to get sick, is to rid our minds of the fear-factor by switching our healthcare belief system. We must first switch from erroneous belief in witches and wizards invoked by enemy and sent after us as cause of illnesses to believing the evidence-based causes of illnesses enumerated in the first section. Once we embrace this fact, then the actions we will take when symptoms present will be in the right direction. Let us use malaria which is very common and kills more people in Nigeria and other sub-Sahara African countries than any other disease as example. Malaria is caused by plasmodium falciparum parasite **(Figure 14)** that resides in the female mosquito salivary gland.

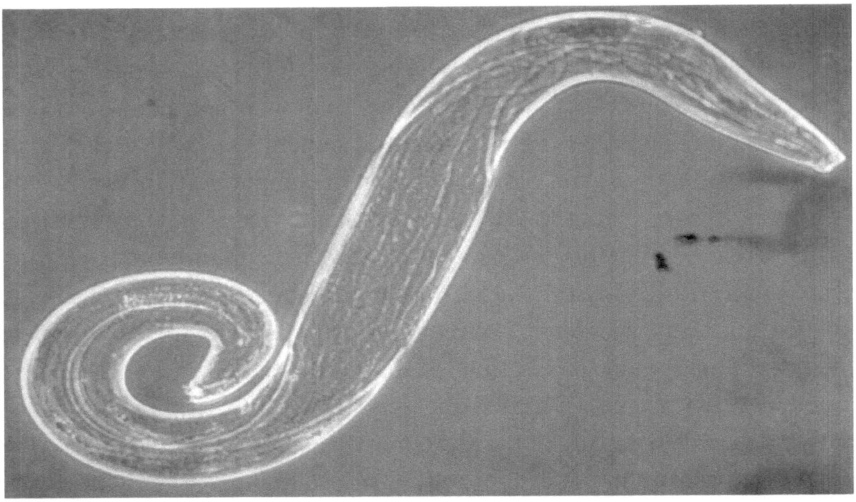

Figure 14

When a female mosquito, acting as a vector (carrier) bites for its blood meal needed to grow her eggs, she injects plasmodium parasite into the bitten victim. The plasmodium parasite heads straight to the victim's liver and later to red blood cells. The disruption and destruction of liver and red blood cells by the parasite results in fever, chills, fatigue, loss of appetite, yellowish skin, and eye (jaundice) seen in a malaria patient. If two individuals were bitten by mosquitos and they develop symptoms as listed above, and one believes that he is being attacked by witches sent by his uncle who is fighting him over his late father's land, he will head straight to a native doctor. The native doctor will ask for eggs, male and female chicken, drinks, money and more. The native doctor will sing all sorts of incantations to confuse him and later gives him bottles of concoction to drink there and some to take home. A few days later he dies. The story does not end here. The falsely accused uncle will forever be labeled a murderer and the seed of enmity sowed by this ignorant belief will forever linger in the family. The other malaria patient who embraced the evidence-based fact that plasmodium parasite causes malaria and goes to a doctor or buys malaria drug from the pharmacy gets cured after few weeks.

Native doctors and so-called prayer warriors exploit the power of what the mind believes and fear-factor to reinforce ignorance-driven healthcare belief system. Native doctors use incantations and prayer warrior uses speaking in the tongue as a means to legitimize their act and confuse their victims. To keep inflow of customers, they capitalize on frightening the public with generational curse as one root cause of their illnesses. They apply the principle of divide and conquer on families by claiming to have seen "visions and prophesies" of one family member being responsible for the sickness and/or death of another family member. The prayer warrior or native doctor deceptively sows seeds of enmity within a family and between families while continuing to collect money for services supposedly rendered from the families. Often the same prayer warrior or native doctor attends to both members of the same family on different days without either having the knowledge they are consulting the same person. The prayer warrior or native doctor uses the information gathered from one family member over the other. As one family member hears the prayer warrior or native doctor repeat what transpired at home with the other family member recounted word-for-word, it legitimizes the prayer warrior's authenticity of possessing supernatural powers. Prayer warriors and native doctors also send their agents as spies after their consultees to gather information. This information is then repeated during consultation, and the consultee on hearing things he or she had said elsewhere will have no doubt in the power the prayer warrior or native doctor claims to possess. Their spies are also sent out to advertise by spreading false rumors of successful healing and deliverances. As a researcher, this author has gone to many of these supposedly powerful healers and found not a shred of credible evidence to their claims. Many of them have their sick family members brought to my attention for help. When I asked why they engage in these deceits and shenanigans, the response is economics; that they have mouths to feed. Here is one example anyone can try. This author has done it successfully several times to prove this point. Get a raffia basket, one egg, piece of red cloth, piece of white cloth, white clay (Nzu), red clay (ughie), and any other fetish you so wish **Figure 15**.

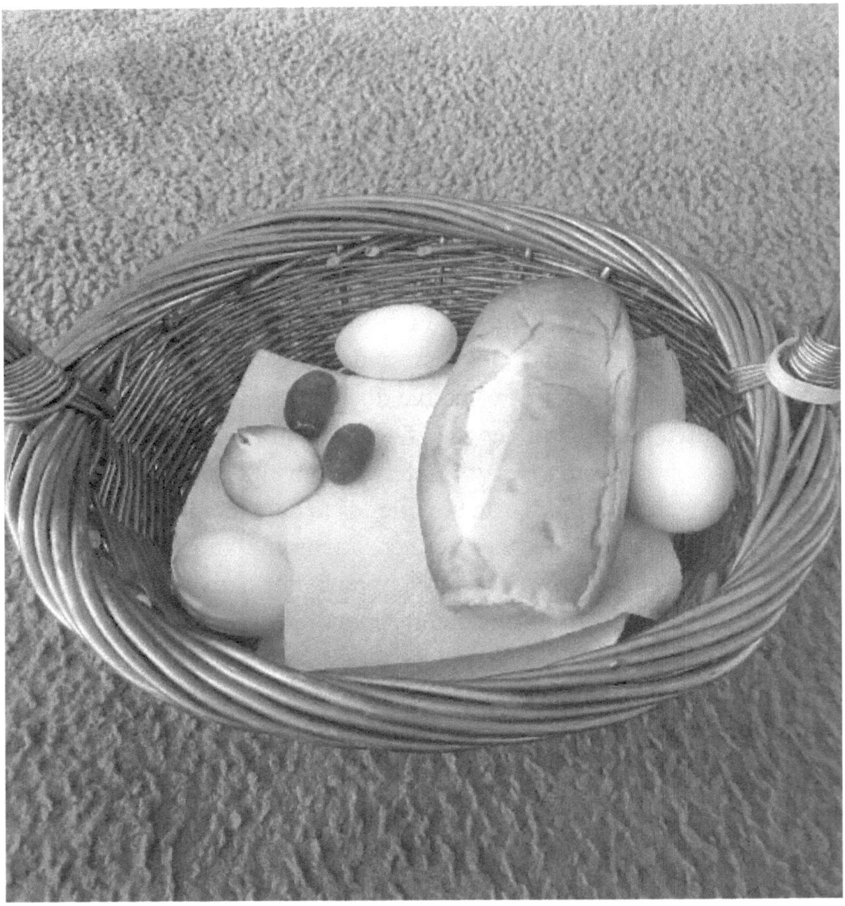

Fig. 15

Load all these items inside the raffia basket. Choose your victim, be sure no one sees you, at night drop it in front of your chosen victim's house. Next morning the house will be deserted, and the entire village will spring into action. There will be as many opinions as the stars in the sky as to who sent it, and reasons for sending it. You may wait to see what items the consulted native doctor or prayer warrior has demanded to use in neutralizing the charm. However, you need to stop the frenzy before your victim could sell all his properties in order to raise funds to appease whatever the native doctor or prayer warrior demanded which usually runs into hundreds of thousands of Naira (Nigeria's local currency). In this case, the witch and wizard are the construct of the fear-factor your mind has ascribed to the basket and its contents. Contrary to the popular saying; seeing is not believing. Instead, the truth is that we interpret what we see within the context of what we believe.

Now, if you have the idea of how your mind takes false information and use it against you, then, you must be careful with what you believe, to whom and what to listen, books you read, and movies you watch. Nollywood movies have done much harm than good in perpetuating the belief in existence of witches and wizards. Most Nollywood production have diabolic scenes in them. Suffice it that these wizardry scenes are intended make-belief fiction, many are not equipped to distinguish them as fiction but belief they are real. It is what you believe that ultimately determines your actions and attitude in all situations. You must begin to control your mind instead of your mind controlling you. You can effectively control your mind only if you verify before you believe, and ensure that only authentic, evidence-based information is stored in your belief system. Fear is said to be an acronym that means; false evidence appearing as real.

If we now believe, what is true, that viruses, bacteria, and other parasites living outside and inside our body, feeding on us for survival, cause damages we regard as illnesses and diseases, then our first line of defense is to reduce or eliminate them from our body and control the sources from which they get to and into our body. Adoption of the popular saying, " prevention is better than cure," but seldom put into practice, is the most cost-effective treatment. Personal hygiene and a clean environment are the first steps one must cultivate in preventing many illnesses. Brushing teeth first thing in the morning, and after each meal, taking a bath at least once a day with clean water and soap, washing hands after using the bathroom, carrying a hand sanitizer on a regular basis, washing cloths regularly, using clean pots to cook, clean plates and spoons to eat, making sure that left over food is properly covered, and properly reheated the next morning before eating are some of many ways to avoid getting sick. Refrigerated foods need to be reheated also before consumption. Many microorganism survive and thrive in very cold conditions, while others thrive in extremely hot conditions.

Remember we live in a competitive world where humans and numerous other organisms compete for both space and food. If your left-over soup, gari, or any food is not covered properly or not covered at all, and a rat gets access to it, eats some of it and defecates or urinates on it, you are into catching one of many disease-causing parasites that rats carry. One deadly such disease carried by rats is Lassa fever which has killed many people in Nigeria over the years. All leftover foods must be covered properly, reheated strongly, and turned over severally while being heated to ensure that heat gets to all parts of the food before it is consumed. Adequate heating will kill most, if not all parasites.

Reference was made earlier in this book to diseases caused by deficiency of micronutrient, such as: vitamins, minerals (i.e., sodium, calcium, zinc, copper, boron, potassium, chromium), phytochemicals, antioxidants, and anti-parasites, found in various natural herbs, vegetables, fruits, and nuts. These micronutrients are in plant leaves, fruits, seeds and roots, and as mineral elements in nature stored by our Creator who knows what is best for good health and long life. They are required in small but crucial amounts, essential for normal biochemical reactions that confer and maintain our body in a healthy state.

Lack of one or more of them result in various illnesses (T**able 3).** There are multiple causes of micronutrients deficiency, such as: inborn deficiency (which can occur when a pregnant mother takes little or no prenatal vitamins), food sources deficient in micronutrients (overuse of farmlands), too young with

immature biochemical pathways unable to extract micronutrient from food sources, too old with weakened biochemical pathways unable to extract micronutrients from food sources, and poor eating habit that excludes sources of micronutrients (junk and processed food).

Nigerians do not eat enough vegetables, fruits, and nuts. For instance, a woman who harvests vegetables, fruits (pineapple, pawpaw, orange), pepper and banana from her farm, takes them to sell in the market, and often, would use the money earned from the sale to buy hair attachments and other outward beautifying items. Then when her gum begins to bleed, and she experiences weakness and fatigue, she runs to a native doctor or prayer warrior for treatment. The native doctor or prayer warrior takes the remaining money she has and stir her in the wrong direction, naming one evil spirit or generational curse responsible for her ailment. Meanwhile, her problem is Vitamin C (ascorbic acid) deficiency, responsible for bleeding gum, and deficiency of Vitamins B12 or Folic acid and/or iron responsible for her general weakness, a symptom of anemia. All these micronutrients she could have easily obtained from eating at least some of the orange and vegetables she harvested and sold in the market.

Clinical Symptoms and Signs of Micronutrient Deficiency

Body Region	Signs	Possible Deficiencies
Skin	Petechiae	Vitamins A, C
	Purpura	Vitamins C, K
	Pigmentation	Niacin
	Edema	Protein, vitamin B1
	Pallor	Folic acid, iron, biotin, vitamins B12, B6
	Decubitus	Protein, energy
	Seborrheic dermatitis	Vitamin B6, biotin, zinc, essential fatty acids
	Unhealed wounds	Vitamin C, protein, zinc
Nails	Pallor or white coloring Clubbing, spoon-shape, or transverse ridging/banding; excessive dryness, darkness in nails, curved nail ends	Iron, protein, vitamin B12
Head/Hair	Dull/lackluster; banding/sparse; alopecia; depigmentation of hair; scaly/flaky scalp	Protein and energy, biotin, copper, essential fatty acid
Eyes	Pallor conjunctiva	Vitamin B12, folic acid, iron
	Night vision impairment	Vitamin A
	Photophobia	Zinc
Oral cavity	Glossitis	Vitamins B2, B6, B12, niacin, iron, folic acid
	Gingivitis	Vitamin C
	Fissures, stomatitis	Vitamin B2, iron, protein
	Cheilosis	Niacin, vitamins B2, B6, protein
	Pale tongue	Iron, vitamin B12
	Atrophied papillae	Vitamin B2, niacin, iron
Nervous system	Mental confusion	Vitamins B1, B2, B12, water
	Depression, lethargy	Biotin, folic acid, vitamin C
	Weakness, leg paralysis	Vitamins B1, B6, B12, pantothenic acid
	Peripheral neuropathy	Vitamins B2, B6, B12
	Ataxia	Vitamin B12
	Hyporeflexia	Vitamin B1
	Muscle cramps	Vitamin B6, calcium, magnesium
	Fatigue	Energy, biotin, magnesium, iron

Table 3

Our bone marrow makes all blood cells including red blood cells. The bone marrow needs two Vitamins, Vitamins B12 (cyanocobalamin) and

B9 (folic acid), and the mineral – iron, to produce red blood cells, which carries oxygen and nutrients to all other cells of the body. Witches, wizards, evil spirits, and generational curse invoked and sent by enemy do not cause Vitamins B12, B9 or iron deficiency that result in disease of anemia. Deficiency of any or all of these micronutrients is due to inadequate consumption of their sources or as a consequence of another existing illness. To avoid developing micronutrient deficiency illnesses, we must eat enough vegetables, especially cruciferous vegetables, fruits, and nuts. (**Figure 16).**

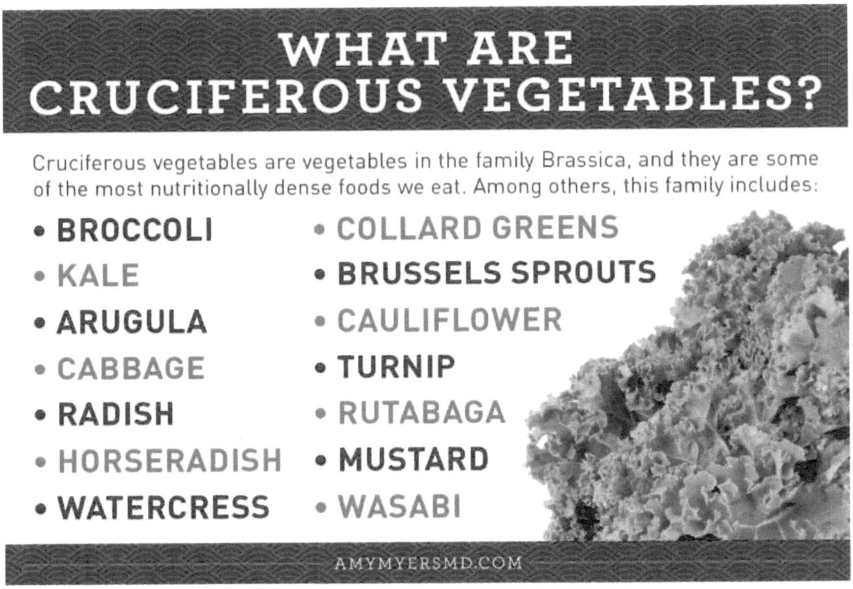

Figure. 16

Eating fruits, nuts, and taking stand-alone vitamins (one vitamin by itself), or multivitamins and multiminerals (a tablet containing all: iron, sodium boron, chromium, magnesium, copper, zinc, potassium) will prevent deficiency of these essential and vital micronutrients. These will provide an adequate number of micronutrients needed to keep up with the demands of the cells' biochemical reactions necessary to achieve and sustain healthy long life.

In developed countries, the most common cause of death is heart diseases. And in Africa it could be the same, or second to malaria, especially in Sub-Saharan African countries. However, African countries are notorious for not keeping good record of diseases, birth, death and other demographic statistics. What is surely evident is that hypertension which results in significant heart disease when not diagnosed on time, not treated adequately, not treated at all or substitution of proven efficacious treatment with herbs and roots with no evidence of efficacy, is common in Africans. It is noteworthy that herbs and roots that have been researched and proven to have health benefits are important integral treatment of various illnesses. The cause of over ninety percent of hypertension is unknown, and current research is pointing to micronutrient deficiencies as potential contributor. It is also speculated that micronutrient deficiencies may account directly for some heart diseases. At least one is well confirmed; deficiency of Vitamin B6 is common in chronic heart failure. What is not clear is the chicken-and-egg paradigm: Vitamins B6, B12 and folate deficiency and heart failure which precedes the other. The jury is still out on the answer. The molecular mechanisms of how micronutrient deficiencies lead to various illnesses is beyond the scope of this book and are better read in various volumes of molecular and cellular medicine. Suffice it to say here that micronutrient deficiency is at the root cause of many illnesses. Eating lots of vegetables, fruits, seeds, and nuts which are natural sources of vitamins and minerals will lead to preventing many illnesses. When there are inadequate natural sources, for the very young and very old, supplementation with micronutrients from commercial sources becomes a necessity.

Type Two diabetes (T2D) is a common illness responsible for lots of premature deaths and permanent disabilities like stroke, heart attack, blindness, and kidney failure. Although science has shown that diabetes, like many other illnesses, has genetic predisposition, it does not imply that a predisposed individual must invariably develop diabetes. In other words, we are not prisoners of our genes. There is a nature-nurture dichotomy interrelationship in disease development, whereby something in the environment must enter or influence the body of a genetically predisposed individual to activate or repress gene(s) responsible for illness. In the case of T2DM, excessive consumption of sugar and sources of sugar; carbohydrates, and hormones produced by fat cells appear to be responsible for inducing the illness. In type One diabetes, it is suspected that an unknown viral infection triggers the immune cells to mistake the cells of pancreas that produce insulin as the triggering virus and destroy them. As a result, the pancreas does not produce insulin anymore for sugar metabolism.

Armed with this information, we can avoid or delay the onset of diabetes by eating less carbohydrates and sugar. For many Africans, carbohydrates which the human body turns into sugar, is staple food. Daily food consumption for some Africans is up to ninety percent carbohydrate. When carbohydrate is broken down, sugar is produced. Sugar is then the ultimate raw material to produce energy the body uses for all activities, both voluntary (walking) and involuntary (breathing). Science has also confirmed that cancer cells cannot survive without sugar. Remember that cancer cells are abnormal cells that continues to divide and grows nonstop, unlike normal cells that grow to maturity and stop growing. A cancer cell is one that refuses to die, but rather continues to multiply and spread. Normal cells reach maturity and die after exhausting their life span. Cancer cells require lots of energy from sugar to sustain their nonstop growth.

Unlike normal cells that has another biochemical pathway of obtaining energy from ketones in the absence of sugar, cancer cells can only use sugar for energy. Ketones are produced by the liver from fats during periods of low or no carbohydrate consumption, fasting or starvation. Therefore, when low or no carbohydrate is being consumed, butter, margarine, coconut oil, and olive oil can be consumed in moderation to supply the liver raw materials to produce ketones. However, for someone overweight or obese, the body can supply the liver with all the fatty oil it needs to produce ketones by breaking down fat stored in fat cells. And the ultimate benefit for the overweight or obese individual is weight loss. Cancer cells can not break down ketones efficiently to obtain energy. As a result, depriving cancer cells of sources of sugar starves them to death. Eliminating sugar and carbohydrates from the diet of a cancer patient is now a frontline natural treatment for all types of cancer. Understandably then, reducing carbohydrate consumption is like using one arrow to kill two birds: diabetes and cancer prevention and treatment, two rampant chronic illnesses wreaking havoc in human population worldwide.

In African culture, treatment of illness is viewed only as taking drugs. However, in reality, prevention, and treatment of the majority of illnesses include for the most part what one does not allow into their body in the first place. Avoiding smoking; (all smokable), excessive alcohol drinking, soft drinks, and commercial fruit juices, which are nothing, but sugar solutions are documented lifestyle practices that protect one from developing various diseases, including cancer. In place of carbohydrates, eat more beans (all types): oil bean (ugba), bread fruit (ukwa), bambara beans (okpa); these are safe healthy sources of plant protein. Plantain (rip and unrip) is safe to be used as fufu. Vegetables, fruits, and nuts must be consumed in abundance. Plantains, especially unripped, can cause constipation. Eating lots of vegetables, fruits and drinking enough water does reduce constipation.

Exercise has been proven as a major contributing factor to attaining and maintaining a healthy long life. Prior to the availability of motorized means of traveling, our ancestors walked on their legs everywhere they went. My grandfather recounted on many occasions how they walked from Mbaise to Port Harcourt, Aba, and other places. These are distances of more than forty miles one way. As recent as early seventies, there was a man who used to carry people on bicycle from Mbaise to Enugu; a journey of about four hours today with vehicle. He outlived all his mates, reaching a ripped age of 93. Daily activities around and within the house is considered exercise. Sweeping, cleaning, hand washing clothes, pounding fufu, climbing and many household chores that involve whole body movements are good exercise. A sedentary lifestyle is a risk for various illness. It is noticeable that affluent women and men with one or more house maids, who hardly do any house chores, ride in cars to everywhere they go, and hardly take a walk, are more prone to become overweight, obese, diabetic, hypertensive, and arthritic to mention the most common ailments affecting this population. Being active is therefore a proven way that contributes to good health and longevity.

One does not need to buy any exercise equipment; walking for thirty minutes a day for most days of the week consistently, is a good start. The key to benefiting from exercise is being consistent. The use of trade mills have been shown to damage knees and does not involve movement of all the muscles. Swimming, playing football (soccer), tennis, basketball, and lifting objects are good exercises that involve movement of most muscles of the body.

Mindfulness, the art of focusing in here-and-now activity with complete exclusion of distractors is a key to avoiding accidents. Mindfulness skills require multiple practices to acquire. Although being careful when climbing, driving, biking, or working with industrial machinery will help prevent accidents, mastering and using mindfulness skills during these activities will reduce accidents significantly. Mindful use of senses, looking and observing the environment, listening attentively, and smelling intensely will help to uncover a potential injury and disease-causing agent lurking in obscure places in an environment. As we are using tiles now in building our house floors, care must be taken to watch for wet floors and sheets of paper on such floors that can slide someone to fall and hit their head on the floor. Some children have died this way. More about this in the case history chapters.

Excessive alcohol drinking has an immediate and late effects of intoxication and withdrawal, respectively. During both times, a drunk driver can cause fatal accident that might kill driver, passengers and/or pedestrians. Alcohol and other psychoactive addictive drugs like marijuana (guuf), heroin, cocaine, and mescaline are well known triggers that lead to mental illnesses such as schizophrenia (craziness), depression, anxiety, and bipolar disorder. Avoiding smoking altogether and drinking excessively are sure ways to mitigate these mental illnesses in a predisposed individual. The only cure for the disease of addiction is never to start smoking or drinking in the first place. We do know that no two individuals are the same, even identical twins. And no two people respond to any drug the same way. Peer pressure is one factor that induces follow-the-crowd, which leads a more vulnerable and less resilient individual to fall victim `of addiction when their peers remain unaffected. Youths must seek out and acquire resistant training to peer pressure. Also, women, though very strong in their own rights, nevertheless, some are easily wooed by their fellow women or men who disguise as friends to indulge in acts they would later regret. There is no suggestion here that men are not vulnerable to peer pressure, however, social research findings show that more men are able to resist friendship coercion. In other situations, both men, women and the youth receive advice from friends, family members and co-workers who do not mean any harm but have little or no knowledge about the condition on which they are advising. There is therefore the need for everyone to question the validity of any information, especially when it relates to health issues. People do out of sympathy mislead others by giving opinion on an issue not familiar to them. And to the recipient, the consequence could become a question of life and death.

Chapter 10

The Right Things to Do When We Are Sick:

First and foremost, you need to be able to identify when you are truly sick or getting sick by knowing what symptoms are. Symptoms are expressible sensations of abnormal changes in any part of your body. Symptoms can be felt, sensed, or seen, and some examples are nausea, cough, fever, pain, headache, dizziness, chills, itching, swollen, diarrhea, constipation, fatigue, weakness, too much, too little or no sleep, secretion from mouth, ear, nose, penis, vagina, anus, and ear. None of these symptoms by itself is a disease entity. Each symptom that occurs alone or in combination with others is nothing but a warning sign that illness is on the way or already present. The norm in Nigeria is for the symptomatic person to go to the chemist, pharmacy, or herbalist to buy drug(s) to treat the symptom(s). Some may go to a pastor or prayer warrior to pray for the symptoms to disappear. There is nothing wrong with treating symptoms whichever way you prefer depending on your health care beliefs, however, when symptom(s) persist more than three days or get worst first day or so, the wisest thing this author recommend is to go straight to a doctor. If there is no doctor within the area or the doctor is not on duty, as is usually the case in most rural areas and villages, a nurse who consults a doctor is an alternative to go to. You are not advised to continue to treat a persisting symptom(s) by buying more of the same drug or other drugs when symptom(s) are getting worst and not improving with symptomatic treatment. Every illness has a widow of opportunity during which it can be arrested and cured, if curable. Continuing self-treatment at home for days or weeks will lead to losing the widow of opportunity for cure. Going on time to a doctor who possesses the specialized knowledge required to evaluate and characterize symptoms will increase the chance of identifying the cause of the symptom(s) and initiate appropriate specific treatment. When you present to a doctor, he or she will assess the symptom(s) by asking you series of questions such as; when did you first see or experience the symptom, is the symptom present all the time or does it come, and go, have you taken any drug, if so, what is the name and dosage of the drug, did the drug help, is there anything that makes it better or worse? If the symptom is cough, the doctor will want to know if you cough out anything. If so, what color and texture. During this assessment known as history gathering, a doctor will ask for past personal illness, family illness, type of work you do, diet, exercise, hobbies, alcohol, and tobacco use as well as social history. Marriage status, level of education, and sexual orientation are all important in aiding to reach accurate specific cause of symptom(s). The doctor will then do a complete physical examination; checking you from head to toe, checking your blood pressure, pulse, and respiration. He will also listen with a statoscope to your lungs, heart, and abdomen for abnormal sounds. It is your presenting symptom(s) that will direct the doctor to which area of the body he has to emphasize his physical examination. However, physical examination involves checking the who body including the brain for mental status.

I hope by now it must be obvious to you that self-treatment of symptom(s) that do not respond to days of treatment will lead to delay of quick and proper identification of true cause of illness. You also must have realized from all the details a doctor must go through to arrive at a true cause of symptoms that neither you, nor your church pastor, co-work, uncle, or friends, all with good intensions and mean no harm, nonetheless feel compelled to render help in the face of persisting symptom(s) and suffering, is equipped with the right knowledge to articulate the symptoms to arrive at the true cause of your symptoms. Such well-meaning loved ones will resort to suggesting you buy more drugs, and in most cases will give you names of drugs they used that was helpful when they were sick. Since many different things can cause the same symptom(s), your loved one's cough might have been due to allergy and yours is due to bacterial infection. Your loved one's fever, running nose and general weakness might be due to viral infection while having the same set of symptoms as you is due to bacterial infection or micronutrient deficiency. You also can ascertain from the lengthy process of history and physical examination a doctor goes through to identify true cause of the symptoms that a laboratory technician or scientist and nurse are not trained in the use of such rigorous processes to pinpoint true cause of symptom(s). With this in mind, I strongly advice that you never refer yourself to a laboratory when you have any symptom(s). The only person to refer you to a laboratory is the same doctor you saw who assessed and examined you and have reasonable suspicion of what might be causing your symptom(s). The doctor will send you to the laboratory with a list of tests he needs results of, to complement his findings from history and examination to arrive at a definitive cause of symptom(s). He may also need to send you for imaging studies like X-ray, magnetic resonance (MRI), Computed tomographic scan (CT-Scan), Ultrasound and any other complementary testing that will enable him reach definitive diagnosis of what caused your symptoms. Under no circumstance should you go to a laboratory on your own for a test without a doctor's referral. The same applies that you do not refer yourself to any or all imaging studies listed above. The duty of a laboratory technician or scientist is to obtain from you the appropriate specimens for the doctor-specified tests, do the tests and send the results to the doctor. The doctor will interpret the results and incorporate them to make a final diagnosis of the cause of symptoms. Only a doctor is trained to give diagnosis. A laboratory technician or scientist, nurse, pharmacist, and you are not trained to give diagnostic causes of illness. Laboratory technician or scientist training is to collect specimens, conduct tests and report results. A nurse interprets, and executes the doctor's orders, monitors a patient and reports observed patient changes to the doctor. A pharmacist dispenses doctor's prescription orders and educates the patient about proper use of the ordered drugs. You should never accept diagnosis and prescription from a laboratory technician or scientist. In the case of nurses, in villages and rural areas where a doctor may not be readily available, a nurse who consults with a doctor can present your symptoms to a doctor who guides her to arrive at a diagnosis. In developed countries, nurses with master's degree known as nurse practitioners and physician assistants can give diagnosis but do so under the supervision of a doctor. The foregoing also applies to X-ray, ultrasound, MRI, and CT-Scan technicians whose job is to follow and conduct doctor's imaging request and report the results to the requesting doctor for interpretation. None of these technicians should be given you diagnosis or prescription for drugs. The doctor can give you prescription for drugs to treat your worrisome symptoms while he is waiting for the results of the laboratory and imaging studies to become available.

When all the results are received back, your doctor will then use information from history, physical examination, laboratory, and imaging studies, to arrive at a definitive diagnosis. Your doctor will sit down with you and explain to you what the cause of your illness is and what treatment you are to receive. Every doctor is a teacher, and this is the teaching moment which is the most important medicine; to explain the risks and causes of your illness and how to avoid recurrence in the future if possible. The doctor will then write a prescription of drugs you need if any, explain none medical treatments if applicable.

The doctor must write legibly the names of all the drugs prescribed. He must go through them one after the other, explaining why he prescribed them, when and how often to take them, take it with or without food, anything like food, drink, or other medicine to avoid while taking them, any side effects and what to do if side effect occurs. A prescriber must provide a phone number to contact him or her if a side effect occurs. A chemist or pharmacist you purchase drugs or micronutrients from, must give these same explanations. When this explanation is not voluntarily provided by a doctor, chemist, pharmacist, nurse, or any other health provider who gives you drug, it is your sole responsibility to demand explanation. It is your only life and the only person to care for it diligently is you. A health care provider is not doing you a favor when he or she is providing your service. You are paying for the service and drugs, as a result, you deserve full disclosure about what you are to put into your mouth. You must know that drugs will cause illness if used inappropriately. Therefore, you must ask questions about things you do not understand about any drugs given to you. And it is your sole responsibility to follow religiously the instructions given to you about the drugs prescribed for you. You must disclose to your doctor or healthcare provider all vitamins, minerals, herbs, and alternative services you are using. You must not stop any drugs prescribed for you on your own. Your doctor is the only one to change, add to or stop your current drugs prescribed for you. All prescribed antibiotics must be taken to completion for the number of consecutive days advised, even if you feel better after taking few of it for less than the days recommended by the prescriber.

Doctor-patient interaction is not a one-way traffic, whereby a patient sits on the receiving end only. You must ask several questions to your doctor. I strongly recommend that when going to visit a doctor you make a list of questions you may ask, take all the drugs you are already using with you and if possible, take a spouse, family member or friend, as a medical-consult companion with you. This medical-consult companion is so important for various reasons, including, but not limited to the following: in case that you are an indigene who does not speak English or pidgin English, the medical-consult-companion will be your interpreter. Also, many medical terminologies do not have vernacular vocabulary (ethnic language) equivalent. This is so pervasive that even the doctors themselves cannot attest to know the vernacular vocabulary equivalent of all parts of the human body. The truth is, not all human body parts have Igbo or any other African local language vocabulary equivalent. This is a significant barrier to realizing adequate doctor-patient communication relationship which affects accurate diagnosis. In these situations, your medical-consult-companion who speaks English can interpret for you, and act as a backup memory who remembers somethings the doctor said that you might forget. Both your illness and being in doctor's office provoke significant anxiety that may cause you mental block resulting in some of the doctor's instructions not registered in your memory.

Chapter 11
Mental Health

Of all health challenges facing Nigeria, no other has such profound stigma and knowledge deficit as mental sickness. And this is because causes and treatment of all mental illness are shrouded in deeply believed superstitions. Nigerians seem not to have the slightest clue of known true causes of various mental illnesses. And evidence of this is obvious by the fact that their loved ones with mental illness litter in market squares like rags **figure. 17**.

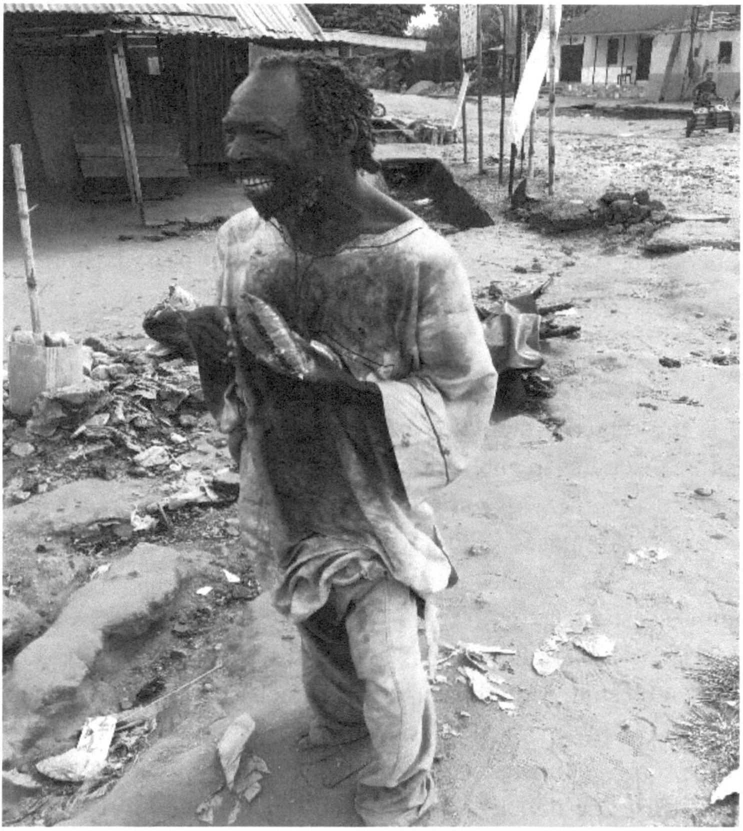

Figure 17

The mentally sick in Nigeria communities are regarded as evil-possessed or has committed one atrocity or the other for which they are infested with a tormenting evil spirit. As a result, little or no help is sought or provided for the mentally sick as they are regarded to be reaping the reward of their sin. Consequently, the mentally sick is left to wonder in market squares. Some mentally challenged, like those whose illness fall into autism spectrum disorder and down syndrome are viewed as sources of curse and shame to the family. Many get murdered by fellow family members, while others are isolated and hidden away within the family out of public sight. The level of abuse experienced by some of these less fortunate members of the family defies humanity.

I have for some decades now flushed out some of these hidden mental challenged individuals in our communities explaining to the families, and the communities evidence-based truth about them. I have dubbed these unfortunate individuals "victims twice;" first born differently for no fault of theirs, and then rejected and subjected to inhumane acts by the same family nature expected to protect them. Families do all these as a result of ignorance, foolish pride, cultural expectation, and firm belief in superstitions handed down from generations past. Historically, in Igboland, before the advent of Christianity, having twins was abomination and mothers of twins were cast out of the community and the twins murdered.

Here is the tragedy, there are available today, affordable and in most cases free resources in public domain that teaches evidence-based known causes and treatment of various mental illnesses. One reason for this tragedy of self-imposed illiteracy is that Nigerians do not read. In fact, it is believed that Black race in general does not read. As a result, there is a popular western saying; "if you wish to hide something from a Black man, put it in a book he will never find it." I personally have done two mini research studies on this supposedly racist saying about Black race. During one of my medical mission trips to Nigeria, I asked teachers of five different secondary schools in which we were doing seminar to name at least one novel or book outside their teaching textbooks they have read in the last five years. I did put out a five-thousand-naira reward for whoever came forward. Amazingly, no teacher claimed the prize. The following year, I bought four novels and put in each a brand new fifty-dollar note. I gave the novels away as a gift to two men and two women. One man and woman I picked at random, and the other man and woman are those who always call me for financial help. Three are high school teachers, and one man works at board of education. During my next trip to Nigeria the following year for another medical mission, I asked the four individuals if they read the novels. Only one woman responded positively. I asked them to bring the books the next day. One lady said her daughter took it to her school, and she would ask for it. They brought the books back separately on different days, and each of the three with unread books were stunned as I pulled out a brand new fifty-dollar note from each of the books and put it in my wallet. The lady who claimed to have read her book confessed that she only flipped through it and a fifty dollar note fell out of it. She told one friend about finding the money. She further said she thought it was mistakenly left in the book. Of course, she cashed and used the money. Surprisingly, the daughter of the other woman who took the book did not read it either.

Although this is a small sample curiosity research, this underscores the truth about the Black race and reading. I have no doubt that the result of expanded research of this type will not be any different. After all, when Nigerians graduate from college, most men read newspapers (mostly politics, soccer, and pool sections), watch soccer, play pool, and Naija-bate, while the women do their hairs and manicure nails. To the best of my knowledge, there is no equipped functioning library anywhere in Nigeria. Comparatively, every town in America has a library, some less than five miles apart, open seven days a week for an average of twelve hours a day and filled up with readers most of the time. A town in America is an equivalent of autonomous community in Nigeria. It is said that readers are leaders. I did not digress, only trying to unveil one of the sources of health illiteracy among Nigerians. Any book is only old to the person who have read it. A book published in the fourteenth century is still a new book to someone who have not read it in the twenty-first century.

Now I am going to mention, but not going into details about known most common mental illnesses and theories explaining their causes and treatment. All the theories proffered to account as causes of different mental illnesses hinge in alteration of the balance, quality and/or quantity of chemical messengers and behavior regulators (hormones and neurotransmitters) produced by human body. Like physical illnesses, environmental factors play a key role in alteration of internal balance of these chemical messengers. As we are going to see, no evil spirit, witches, wizards, or voodoo has been uncovered by science research as the cause of any of the mental illnesses.

The common denominator of the evidence-based causes of all mental illnesses like physical illnesses is the nature and nurture dichotomy, in which there is an interaction between an environmental, and natural factors to cause illness. In the case of mental illnesses, the chemical messengers in human body; hormones and neurotransmitters are altered in such a way that when there is a deviation from the absolute critical amount required for normal expression of mood, perception or feeling, abnormal behavior is expressed. In other words, when one or more of these chemical messengers is/are deficient or excess in the amount required to affect their nature determined normal activity, the affected individual exhibits a behavior that is out of his or her cultural norm. This deviation from acceptable cultural norm is what is known as mental illness. I will mention the names of some of the involved chemical messengers as we discuss specific mental health disorders.

The most common mental illnesses worldwide are anxiety disorders, depression, Schizophrenia, Bipolar, Autism spectrum disorder, personality disorder and substance use disorder. Anxiety disorders are perhaps the most common illnesses in the entire world. Examples of anxiety disorder are panic attacks, general anxiety disorder, obsessive compulsive disorder, phobic disorders, social anxiety disorders and post traumatic disorders. Even when anxiety does not rise to a level of sickness, it is present in almost all situations of life. When someone is diagnosed with any other illness, there is always an anxiety component that accompanies it. The intensity of anxiety experienced in the company of another diagnosed illness is proportionate to how the illness is viewed as a threat to life by the sick person and the community. For instance, a diagnosis of cancer, of which science does not yet have a significant solution to cure, is generally viewed as a life-threatening situation in all cultures and it provokes the most intense anxiety in all countries. Winning the lottery, facing examination, passing examination, getting married, getting divorced, expecting a child, buying a new car or house, all do provoke a certain level of anxiety. In need, as in plenty, there is anxiety. No wonder then, the Creator of life, in His manual of life, which Christians hijacked as their own, and named Bible, admonished that the living should not be anxious about anything. He, being all knowing, knew how pervasive and debilitating anxiety could be. This author believes that the Bible is a living manual for all humans, Christians, and none Christians.

Functionally, humans are dependent on chemicals; our internal function uses hormones and neurotransmitters to cause all activities, from movement, breathing, thinking, perception, memory storage, retrieving memory to virtually all human activities. And these internal chemicals respond to external factors that act as stimulators, cues, and triggers to launch them into action. Since the interaction of internal neurotransmitter and external trigger is very complex, an alteration of any kind at any or multiple levels of the process will result in abnormality. The three known neurotransmitters that mediate anxiety are Serotonin, Gama-amino butyric acid (GABA) and Norepinephrine. Neither these neurotransmitters nor their external triggers are a witch, wizard, or evil spirit. However, if you are afraid of someone who you believe is diabolic, seeing the person or mere hearing his name can trigger an outpour of these neurotransmitters to induce anxiety and panic attack. The longer the thinking, feeling and fear of perceived impending doom lingers, the more intense the anxiety. Intense lingering anxiety of several months to years has been linked to physical heart disease. This falls into another group of illnesses known as psychosomatic illness. Psychosomatic means disease of the mind that affects, and results in physical body illness. Mind over the body.

Schizophrenia is the mental illness Nigerians regard as craziness. It is characterized by hallucination (perception of unreal sensation) and paranoid (excessive or irrational distrust or suspicion of others). An affected individual can describe seeing, hearing, smelling, and touching things that are not real which others around him cannot perceive. Other characteristics of craziness is delusion, having bizarre thoughts, and disorganized speech. Dopamine and Serotonin are two neurotransmitters research evidence shows that their alteration plays a key role in causing schizophrenia. Too much dopamine in certain parts of the brain causes over stimulation which results in difficulty in thought processes, reality orientation, feelings, concentration, and behavior. Recent evidence has demonstrated that alteration in amount of serotonin in certain areas of brain contributes to development of schizophrenia.

Autism spectrum disorder includes Autism, Asperger Syndrome, and pervasive developmental disorder. Affected children usually appear normal at birth and continue to develop appropriately until just about or from two years old, they begin to slow down and regress from gains already made in development. They begin to lose interest in people and focus interaction mainly with inanimate objects. They avoid facial contact and interaction with people. The word spectrum means that no two individuals with autism are alike, and each has his or her own unique strength and deficit. However, all have poorly developed social skills, expressive and receptive communication skills, and restrictive and repetitive patterns of behavior.

There are several theories being proposed with several environmental substances and conditions being suspected as triggers to ASD development. Generally accepted is that an environmental trigger causes disruption in the normal development of the neurons that produce various neurotransmitters. The three neurotransmitters evidence shows their alteration as being most contributory is Gama amino butyric acid (GABA), Glutamate and Serotonin. Also involved are Catecholamine and Acetylcholine neurotransmitters.

Depression is a very common and serious mental illness. Although all mental illnesses are serious and require immediate recognition and treatment, depression needs extra special attention in that it is more prone to lead to suicide than any other. In the medical community, there are many types of depression that we are not going to discuss here. Our discussion here refers to the most serious known major depressive disorder. Whereas it is normal for someone to feel sad and have low mood sometimes, especially when one is struck with adverse life events like death of loved one, loss of job, divorce, low on or no cash, it is abnormal when the feeling of sadness persists for several weeks and even months. Most common symptoms of depression are loss of interest in activities one used to enjoy, loss of appetite or increase in appetite, weight loss, or gain unrelated to dieting, lack of sleeping or sleeping too much, loss of energy or increased fatigue, increase in purposeless activities; slow speech, pacing around, feelings of worthlessness, hopelessness, and helplessness, and making death or suicide gestures. Postpartum depression is common but not easily recognized and occurs in women after child delivery. The three neurotransmitters implicated in causing depression are Serotonin, Norepinephrine and Dopamine. It is believed that alteration in these three neurotransmitters by a trigger is responsible for causing depression. I must point out here that none of these neurotransmitters which when in balance result in normal mood, and when unbalanced result in altered mood and behavior known as depression is a witch, wizard, or evil spirit. It is normal to grief the death of a loved one for a while. However, when grief lasts more than six months to a year, and the grieving individual exhibits most of the characteristics of major depression listed above, it is no more grief, but disease of depression.

It is not unusual for recently bereaved individual to see apparitions of the diseased one or see him in dreams almost all nights in the first few months following his death. It is the perpetual preoccupation and thinking of the deceased loved one that creates the illusive apparitions such as seeing the figure of the diseased pass swiftly in seconds. In these situations, it is the preoccupation with the deceased that alters the balance of the activities of the neurotransmitters to create apparitions. Intense fear induced by seeing apparitions can lead to intense anxiety, panic attacks, increased blood pressure, heart rate and abnormal palpitation of the heart. The most important thing to watch for in someone depressed is suicide threats. Never take such threats lightly especially when plans to carry it out is being voiced or unusual behaviors like self-isolation is present.

Bipolar disorder is a mental disorder formerly known as manic depression. It is characterized by extreme mood swings of emotional highs (mania or hypomania) and then lows (depression). When in mania or hypomania (less mania but above normal mood) phase, affected individual feels euphoric, full of energy, irritable and may get involved in risky behavior. When he shifts to depression phase, he feels sad, hopeless, helpless, loss of interest and pleasure in activities previously enjoyed. Expert scientists have not uncovered the complete cause of bipolar mood swings. However, the advances made so far indicate that problems with the wiring of brain circuits and neurotransmitter chemical messengers are partly involved. Dopamine, Serotonin, and norepinephrine neurotransmitters are the three culprits thought to have the problem that leads to bipolar disorder. Again, I will point out the fact that these neurotransmitters are not witches, wizards, or demons inside the human brain. Science has clearly identified several chemical messengers produced by the brain cells and responsible for affecting human activities through alteration of moods and emotions.

Using a car engine for analogy, when fuel, brake fluid and engine oil are running very low to empty, their respective specific light indicators come on to warn the driver. The driver will have to do something before it hits empty. It is the same in the human brain and the rest of his body. The chemical messengers: neurotransmitters and hormones on which the smooth functioning of human mood and emotions depend must be maintained within a specific critical amount for normal function. An alteration that makes a chemical messenger to be less or more of the critical normal amount required for normal behavior will disrupt normal function and result in mental disorder. Out of ignorance, superstitious beliefs in the myths of witches, wizards, evil spirits, and demons still lingers among Nigerians as causes of mental illness.

Personality disorder is an engraved pattern of feeling, thinking, and behaving that is out of range from the expectations or norms of a culture and causing difficulties in interpersonal relationships and in society. These are subtle but devastating to those in contact with affected individuals. They do have a spectrum of expression from mild to severe cases. There are several types of personality disorder: paranoid, schizoid, schizotypal, antisocial, borderline, histrionic, narcissistic, avoidant, dependent, and obsessive-compulsive.

Suspiciousness is the dominant feature of paranoid, schizoid, schizotypal and antisocial personality disorders. Those with borderline, histrionic, and narcissistic personality disorders tend to be emotional. Avoidant, dependent, and obsessive-compulsive personality disorder individuals are mostly anxious.

It is thought that problems with one or more neurotransmitters is responsible for different personality disorders. The number of neurotransmitters produced in human body is many and each fall into eight main groups; amino acids, gastrotransmitters, monoamines, trace amines, peptides, purines, catecholamine, acetylcholine, and anandamide that do not fall into any of the above seven groups. Naming specific neurotransmitters and their involvement in specific personality disorders is beyond the scope of this book. Our take home from here is that several decades of careful scientific study of the human brain and body has discovered the chemical messengers of which alteration in their normal activity results in behaviors that are off cultural expectations referred to as personality disorders. This evidence therefore should replace the unsupported beliefs in demons, witches, wizards, and evil spirits as responsible for mental illness.

Substance use disorder also known as drug addiction is a disease of the brain which alters behavior and results in inability of the affected individual to control the use of legal or illegal drugs. Some of the drugs involved are:

Alcohol, Marijuana (**Guuf**), Codeine, Valium, Librium, Tramadol, Cocaine, Amphetamine, Heroine, Vicodin, Oxycodone, Morphine and several more. And more recently; water seed or drop (**mkpuru miri**) a concoction of various mood altering legal and illegal drugs innovated in Nigeria is recking havoc among the youth.

These drugs are chemical molecules and share certain structural features with the natural brain chemical messengers known as neurotransmitters. Acting as disrupters, these drugs alter the production and use of natural neurotransmitter that leads to the user losing ability to control use. In many cases drug addiction results in permanent disability of the addict, rendering him nonproductive. Drug addiction is a mental illness growing at exponential rate among the youths in Nigeria. Drug addiction is the most common cause of school dropouts and loss of productivity. Sadly, the only cure for drug addiction is, not to start use in the first place. It is obvious in the case of substance use disorder; the cause is known to be identifiable drugs and not attributed to demons, witches, and wizards. But wait, Nigerians still label marijuana addicts as demon-possessed or bewitched by enemies.

Lifestyle Changes to Achieve Healthy Living

Change of any form is always difficult to embrace by either an individual or society. Previous chapters have shown that there is an imminent need for us to believe in the evidence-based findings of true causes of illnesses if we must live healthily and longer. We are now to make the same change the medieval residents of western countries made when bacteria were proven to cause infections, and antibiotics were discovered to cure it. We have a similar situation today with scientific evidence showing that the root cause of noninfectious illnesses such as heart diseases, diabetes, hypertension, and cancers responsible for majority of premature deaths are what we eat, drink, inactivity or lack of exercise and other risky lifestyles. And the root cause of infections are viruses, bacteria, worms, and other parasites. Evidence has it that abnormal alteration of the immune system function due to our lifestyle and influence of environmental factors, of which some are not amenable to our control result in such diseases as allergies and autoimmune diseases.

Science also has shown that all mental illnesses result from abnormal alteration of natural neurotransmitters by environmental triggers, many of which are not known yet.

Stress, which can be emotional, psychological, spiritual, or physical, has long been shown to be a major risk factor that triggers some physical and mental illnesses. Neither science nor any other study modality has shown that witches, wizards, voo doos, or evil spirits cause any physical or mental illness. These mythical concepts are nothing but a construct of the human mind from internalized erroneous beliefs.

When the mind is rid of mythical beliefs and filled with evidence-based facts, behavior and action will change. And this is what we must do now, to drop previously believed myths about risks and causes of illnesses, replacing them with the evidence-based new information presented here, and found on the internet and many texts. Although change of all form is difficult to embrace, but when the change that must be made involves life and death, there should be no other option, and all debates and denials to justify continuing such lifestyle that indisputable evidence has shown will ultimately lead to premature death must be dropped. Anyone who has worked in an addiction treatment center or hospital must be familiar with patients who would acknowledge that for several decades they were aware that chronic heavy cigarette smoking would lead to lung cancer. But they continued to smoke, despite possession of this life-saving information, only to stop smoking the moment they were diagnosed with lung cancer. Unfortunately, stopping at this point is very late, and for many, premature death is inevitable. In the early 80's I was involved in campaigning for eliminating cigarette smoking in hospitals and all public areas in Chicago and entire United States of America. I even authored a poem for my smoking patients.

Beloved Smoker

Thou should stop smoking,
Your gains smoking is
very temporary; suffering
very permanent

You, an adult; truth about
smoking, very little you know.
The little you know, you believe not.

Thou should stop, for each puff takes
you, even closer to an earlier
grave. Earlier grave, after
most painful, agonizing
illness.

Yes, some dangers about smoking,
you heard, but knowledge
not applied to improve living
is a wasted Knowledge.

Today there is no smoking in hospitals and all public areas in America. Some establishments have set out signs that depicts the distance away from their building where one can smoke. Airports and other public areas like restaurants have designated enclosed smoking areas. It took hard work of intense persistent campaign to accomplish as the giant multibillion-dollar cigarette manufacturers mounted seemly formidable opposition to derail the stop-smoking in public spaces campaign.

Chapter 12
Diet and Nutrition

It is universally believed from currently best available evidence that the most external risks for most illnesses responsible for premature death are what we eat and drink, how much we eat and drink, how often we eat and drink, lack of exercise, sedentary lifestyle, and persistent stress. Apart from natural laws promulgated by the Creator, such as the Sun must rise from the East and set in West daily, most things are dynamic and not static. Even new scientific findings do lead to more research that yield results nullifying previously believed findings. Even societal cultures and traditions are not static, but dynamic, whereby civilization and technology constantly alter previously practiced cultures and held traditions.

Like many other Africans, many Nigerians have carbohydrates as their staple food, and it constitutes more than eighty percent of daily food consumed. Carbohydrates in the form of table sugar, rice, yam, cocoyam, potatoes, cassava, gari, three-leaf yam, bread, biscuits, chim-chim, bons, kpof-kpof and various flour products are eaten several times daily. These different carbohydrate forms will be degraded to the final smallest molecule; glucose, which then enters inside the cell with the help of insulin produced by the pancreas. In the cell, glucose is turned into the energy that powers all body activities. But, because the sugar produced is in excess of what the body needs at any given time, it becomes detrimental to the body in a way that results in diabetes, hypertension, high cholesterol, and cancers among other diseases.

It is my speculation that our ancestors ate more carbohydrates and less fruits, vegetables, and nuts because carbohydrates filled the stomach and provided much needed energy for farm work and other physical activities. There were no machines to help in all the activities, including mobility. They walked hundreds of miles to their destinations. As a result, the large amount of carbohydrates they consumed was burned for energy needed for the physically demanding daily activities. However, for us, there are all sorts of machines to help with household chores, mobility, and other work activities. A common blender in the kitchen eliminates pounding pepper with mortar and pestle which sapped lots of human energy. A carpenter has many tools at his disposal today that limit the use of human energy. We build houses now with blocks and not with mud, and the energy spent to mold blocks is much less than the use of bare feet to mix mud for building. I hope you get the idea that we need less energy and therefore less carbohydrates today than our ancestors. The excess glucose formed from the excess carbohydrate eaten and not needed since we are spending less energy is converted to fat. Our body is perhaps the most sophisticated refinery the Creator made. It can interconvert molecules. The body has both current and savings account in the form of energy to expend now and energy stored for future use. Energy to spend now formed from glucose is known as adenosine triphosphate (ATP) and energy stored for future us is fat. It is obvious that our population is heavier today because there is more food available, we eat more and use less energy, hence excess glucose is stored as fat. It is estimated that up to 25% of Nigerians are overweight or obese. It is important to know that carbohydrates provide mainly calories for energy but little or no micronutrients essential to maintain a healthy body. Micronutrients are essential coenzymes of the biochemical reactions for the immune cells production of their weapons of mass destruction needed to destroy parasitic invaders and cancer cells.

The recommendation then, and the change we must make is to eat less carbohydrates and more plant-based foods. Think of it this way, anything that grows below the ground, rice and corn must be eaten in a limited quantity and less often. Plant-based foods available for Nigerians are all types of beans and products of beans like akara, moi-moi, and okpa, oil bean, bread fruit, lots of various vegetables, fruits, and nuts. We do not need to eat to fill our stomach, but rather to consume those items containing phytonutrients essential for body growth, repair, enhancement, and support of the immune system. And we should not eat any food or drink any drink anymore because we were raised with it, or because of its taste, smell, look, availability, even when free. Rather, we should eat according to evidence-based information as to what the phytonutrient (phytochemical) content of the food and what it can do to confer healthy living.

Chapter 13
Exercise and Physical Activities

The importance of what we eat run neck-and-neck with exercise or physical activity in determining health and life span. Several research over the years have produced the same results showing both diet and exercise as the keys to achieving healthy living, reduced risks for illnesses and long-life span. Healthy diet and moderate level of exercise also have been confirmed to be the fabrics of aging gracefully. The third important element in addition to healthy diet and exercise to determine healthy living, aging gracefully and long-life span is stress reduction or management.

Exercise or physical activity is important because of its role in energy expenditure. We have discussed the fact that energy not expended is stored in the body as fat from which the body taps into when faced with starvation or reduced food intake during intentional religious fasting or famine. And when the stored fat is not utilized, it becomes a liability that results in sickness. Fat cells, like other cells of the body, are alive and active. Fat cells produce known hormones that are detrimental to our health. In an overweight or obese person, these bad hormone reck havoc to normal cells, hence overweight and obesity are well known harbingers for various chronic diseases. This is so life threatening that a separate specialist field known as obesity medicine that focuses on weight loss programs has evolved.

There are four types of exercise, and each is necessary and complement others to achieve the healthy goal. Aerobic exercise such as running, jogging, brisk walking, swimming, basketball, volleyball, football, house chores; mowing lawn, farming, swiping, racking, and mopping are all important. Aerobics are the type of exercise most people in Africa do, usually as part of their daily activities of living. Especially in the rural areas, walking and house chores constitute the major exercise done. There are no gyms or time set aside for exercise. It is also evident that premature deaths in the rural population is predominantly due to infectious diseases and injuries than from diabetes, high blood pressure and high cholesterol. However, this is also changing since the rural population began to eat processed food and ride on motor bikes (**Ina aga or Okada**) and tricycle (**Keke na Pepe**). The rural population does not walk as much as before, uses wheelbarrows to carry loads, and there are bore holes available now in most areas, as a result, children do not have to walk miles to fetch water from rivers anymore.

All these improvements that limit use of human energy for all activities are welcomed but carry the negative effect of less human energy expenditure. In addition, with the availability of television and Nollywood, people sit long hours at a time watching movies and piling up weight. Aerobic exercise targets and improves the heart, lungs, and circulatory system, increases good cholesterol, decreases bad cholesterol, risk of heart attack, diabetes type two, high blood pressure and stroke. A study of 1.4 million people in America and Europe and another large study of 660,000 people shows that those who did aerobic exercise of 150 minutes per week had a 31% less risk of dying in the next 14-years period than those who did not do exercise. A moderate intensity aerobic exercise of 150 minutes per week divided into 30minutes each day for five days is enough to confer good health. 75 minutes of vigorous aerobic exercise per week will confer the same health benefit as moderate activity of 150 minutes per week. The key is being consistent and doing it routinely. The main complication of aerobic exercise is developing joint problems. You must avoid high impact activities like jumping. For all exercises, at the initial stage, you must start low and go slow.

Strength exercise is another type of exercise and includes weightlifting, push-ups, crunches, working muscles using resistances, pushing against objects, pull-ups, and using weight machines. This type of exercise increases lean muscle mass, bone density, metabolism, helps in weight loss, burns more calories, and lowers risk of injury. It also improves the body's use of insulin and reduce blood sugar level. You can do this type of exercise at least two days a week. Work on major muscle groups; legs, hips, back, chest, abdomen, shoulders, and arms. You can do eight to twelve repetitions of activity per muscle group. Do not do the same muscle groups for two consecutive days to avoid injury.

Balance exercise increases the ability to control and stabilize the body's position. This is very useful exercise for older adults because as humans age, proprioception; the ability to know where we are relative to space around us gets worse. Some examples of balance exercise are shifting body weight side to side, standing on one foot, walking heel to toe, using balance board or stability ball, doing tai chi, yoga, or Pilates. Balance exercise prevents falls, reduce risk of lower extremities injury, and improves proprioception.

There is no limit to how many times one can do balancing exercise. You can do 3 to 6 times per week with four per session for eleven to twelve weeks to improve balance. The main risk of this exercise is fall. You must have something next to you, you can hold onto when off balance to avoid fall. Older adults need to have someone in their company when doing balancing exercises.

Flexibility exercise is to stretch muscles and improve the range of motion of the joints. It is of two types; static stretching which is muscle stretch without movement and dynamic stretching which combines stretching with movement. Examples of static stretching are stretching hamstring muscles by sitting on the ground with legs straight and leaning forward, calves stretching by stepping forward with one leg and shifting your weight toward the front leg and thigh muscle stretching by bending one leg back toward your buttocks and holding onto your foot.

Examples of dynamic flexible exercise is raising your knee toward your chest and holding onto the shin, and then bringing your leg down. Do the same with the opposite leg.

This can be done standing still or walking. Ankle stretching involves raising one foot up slightly off the ground, keeping leg straight and flex foot with toes pointing up. Repeat with the opposite foot. Arm swinging is done by stretching both arms in front of you with palms facing down. Then walk forward and swing your arms together to right with your left arm crossing your chest and swing to the left with right arm crossing your chest. Continue walking and repeating several times in the opposite directions. Arm circles is accomplished by holding the arms outside ways parallel to the floor. Do arm circles in both clockwise and anticlockwise directions several times until you are not able to do the next circle. Flexibility exercises improve flexibility of joints, reduce risk of injury, and reduce lactic acid in muscles. There is no limit to how many times these can be done in a week.

All these four exercises can be done in one exercise routine in one day, using flexibility and stretch exercise as warm up for aerobic type and finishing with balance exercise. You can design your own combination sequence of the four and being mindful not to overdo either one to avoid injuries. Thousands of free videos of all four types of exercises can be seen on Youtube.

Chapter 14
Stress Reduction

Before delving into various techniques or strategies for reducing stress, I would like to emphasis that the major determinant of good health, prevention of illness, aging gracefully and long life is what we eat, how physically active we are, and how we handle stress. Stress is a fact of life and not avoidable by any known means. However, it can be managed effectively to minimize its adverse contribution to illness and premature death. Although there are formal strategies that help manage stress, Africans use these strategies informally without consciously applying them to reduce stress. Unlike in developed countries where there are gyms, spas, tract fields and public swimming pools built with stress reduction in mind, it is only recently that such amenities are springing up in some African cities for commercial purposes. However, Africans do get involved in various stress reduction strategies on their daily routine activities.

The most utilized stress reduction strategies by Africans (prayer, singing and dancing) are interwoven as activities of their religion not necessarily thinking of them as stress management activities. Most Nigerians must go to church or mosque on a regular basis. Although their intent is to go worship and pray but may not be aware that it does reduce spiritual, emotional, psychological, and physical stress. Like all other stress reduction techniques, the religious activities of prayer, singing, and dancing do cause the release of natural pain soothing and pleasure inducing neurotransmitters (dopamine, enkephalin, endorphin and oxytocin). Paying tithes or giving offering in the church also invokes release of these pleasure neurotransmitters. Giving and caring for someone as well as showing gratitude for help rendered to you are all subtle but important stress reduction techniques. All practicing Christians must be familiar with the admonition in the manual of life that states; it is better to give than to receive. Exercise is another stress management strategy which among Africans is usually not formally done separately but linked to daily chores and sport activities. Cleaning the house, working on the farm, washing clothes with hands, pounding fufu or pepper, mopping the floor and other daily house chores, all of which can be combined with singing and/or listening to music are all stress reducing. Singing, listening to music, and dancing, all of which can be done alone or in combination are important stress management techniques. Reading and writing are very soothing stress reducing activities. Laughing aloud, watching comedies and selected movies are important stress management techniques. Comedies that provoke laughing are much more dependable to provoke release of pleasure neurotransmitters than some movies that do provoke stress. You must be careful with movies which you may not know their content beforehand as many can provoke stress. In my estimate, more than sixty percent of Nollywood movies are loaded with juju and cultic scenes that reinforce belief in witches, wizards, evil spirits, and demons.

As discussed previously, the memory of these movies continues to replay and sustain release of those stress provoking hormones and neurotransmitters. It is therefore important that you must be cautious of what movies you watch and what you believe. Mindfulness, deep breathing, and guided imagery are used separately or in combination to reduce stress. For those who have access to YouTube on the internet you can search for anyone of these stress reduction modalities to view how they are done. Other stress management techniques which can be learned from the YouTube are Yoga, Tai chi, Tai gong, massage, and several other techniques of the Asian origin. Going to spas and massage salons are well documented stress limiting treats to yourself. Reaching out to talk to someone you trust discussing positive uplifting issues and not negative gossips is stress reducing. All sport games done in moderation does elicit pleasure and pain 53soothing neurotransmitters. Challenging your mind with creative and innovative thinking in writing, designing, cooking, and even working on creating a local stress reduction strategy is stress reducing. Going on vacation away from where you are too familiar with and being adventurous is soothing to the body and mind. African culture does not include taking time out or going on vacation to relax and reduce stress and tension of everyday works of life. This must change for Africans to achieve healthy long life.

Chapter 15
The Truth about Healing

The World Health Organization defined health as "state of complete physical, mental, and social well-being and not merely the absence of disease or infirmity." Healing means restoration to normalcy. I would like to touch on one misconception of Africans about illness and healing. Africans, like every other human on earth dislike change, and embrace novel ideas and projects very reluctantly. When an African is sick, he expects nothing short of returning fully to his initial healthy condition. The concept of acute and chronic illness is not known and appreciated. However, the reality is that the course of some illnesses is acute, and they can be cured or healed outrightly, returning the sick to the very normal state of health he or she was in before the sickness. Most acute illnesses are infections or body injury in nature, caused by viruses, bacteria, and other parasites such as malaria, gonorrhea, candidiasis, pneumonia, ulcer, typhoid, and accidents, respectively.

However, if a disease that has an acute course is not caught early enough and treated appropriately, it can lead to permanent complication that becomes chronic. This underscores the importance of seeking medical care as early as symptoms are noticed. Chronic diseases are those that cannot be cured and has a life-long course. Chronic illnesses are usually non-infectious such as diabetes, hypertension, asthma, Parkinson disease, multiple sclerosis, rheumatoid arthritis, osteoarthritis and many more. Whereas chronic diseases are not healed or cured outright, they are not necessarily death sentence as they can be managed with necessary lifestyle changes and specific drugs to avoid potential complications and enable the individual live long life. Emerging evidence is pointing to the possibility of cure of some non-infectious chronic illness if they are caught early and appropriate treatment instituted.

However, when it comes to cure and healing, no drug heals any illness; the body heals itself. Protecting the body and supplying it with the necessities to heal itself when infected or injured is the sole natural work of the immune system. The immune system comprises several specialized cells that work cooperatively to heal the body. All manufactured drugs and modalities used in treatment only help the immune system to do its healing work. When an individual is shot and a bullet lodges in the thigh for example, a healthcare provider will first try to stop bleeding and clean the bullet entrance with antiseptics to prevent bacteria and other parasite infection. A surgeon will operate to extract the bullet. If the bullet is extracted, the surgeon will do the best possible to approximate the tissues together and close the wound. The body's blood clotting mechanism began its work even before the healthcare provider reaches the wounded individual. The clotting mechanism is the one that eventually stops bleeding. The band aid covering over the wound only protects the wound from being contaminated or infected while the immune cells do the healing of sealing and repairing the wound. Antibiotics and tetanus injections all work to prevent infection and do not by themselves effect healing. The expert healer-cells that make up the immune system will use micronutrients; vitamins and minerals of which Vitamin C is highly crucial to heal the wound. Vitamin C functions as a co-enzyme in the production of collagens which are protein fibers that close wounds. Various other vitamins, minerals, and amino acids function as co-enzymes in different biochemical pathways for wound healing.

If the bullet lodged in such location that it is not extractable, the immune cells will heal the wound and wall off the bullet. The need for you to eat a balanced diet rich in vegetables, fruits, seeds, and nuts from where phytonutrients are derived for healing cannot be over emphasized. Perhaps you have noticed that wounds on diabetic patients heal slowly or not at all, for which amputation of toes and extremities must be performed to save life. This is because excess sugar in the body impedes the work of immune cells in healing by damaging blood vessels, in effect, reducing blood flow that contains nutrients and oxygen essential for immune cells to provide healing. For this reason, diabetic patients must be careful not to injure themselves. Antibiotics can kill bacteria and antivirus can kill viruses, but their lifeless remains are still foreign to the body provoking immune reaction that ultimately eradicates them. If not, the lifeless remains of killed bacteria and viruses would perpetually provoke another illnesses. In effect, the immune system only hills using natural resources from diets and supplements. All man-made products function to aid the immune system do its natural duty of healing the body.

Within the last decade, and since the advent of internet and other social media, the medical and pharmaceutical profession is not able to dictate for the public all about healthcare. Much of the information previously available only to the healthcare industries are now in the public domain. Consequently, there is public realization that synthetic drugs, surgery, chemotherapy, and radiotherapy do not cure but aid the body to heal itself when supplied with adequate and complete natural products. Now, there is a rapid growth in the natural healing industry where vitamins, minerals, herbs, and essential oils are being used successfully to heal illnesses. Many allopathic doctors (medical doctors) are buying into the role of natural herbs, alternative and complementary treatment modalities for healing. These medical doctors who are trained in natural healing are known as integrative doctors. Integrative means that they use a combination of prescription drugs, natural products, alternative and complementary modalities to provide individualized holistic treatment. For instance, a patient with low back pain (a common illness worldwide) who goes to an integrative doctor, may be asked to apply warm towel at the back or heated stone wrapped in a towel (non-medical treatment), apply shea butter **(okwuma or ori),** use turmeric and black pepper as cooking spice, or take turmeric capsules or tablets, fish oil (natural products), do exercise, massage, acupuncture (complementary modalities), acupressure, use tylenol, ibuprofen, tramadol and injection of steroids. The integrative doctor can recommend these options in various combinations and may eventually recommend surgery. A non-integrative medical doctor can recommend all the things the integrative doctor recommended in various combinations but will not include shea butter, turmeric, fish oil and acupuncture in his list. When it comes to cancer, neither surgery, chemotherapy nor radiotherapy provides complete healing. Both chemotherapy and radiotherapy which cost thousands to millions of Naira kill both normal and cancer cells hence their numerous debilitating side effects. It is only the immune cells that are naturally equipped to distinguish normal cells from cancer cells. Immune cells will destroy cancer cells. Even when chemotherapy, and radiotherapy kill cancers and antibiotics kill bacteria, the debris of dead cells accumulates and can cause diseases of its own. It is the specialized scavenger immune cells that clear these dead cells and invader debris. To keep the immune system at its optimal functioning capacity is a task that must be done to sustain health and prevent premature death.

Chapter 16
True Life Cases

In this section, this author presents some actual cases he worked on in Nigeria over the years, selecting one outstanding case from different disease category. To maintain the privacy of the patients, fictious initials, rather than the real name initials of each patient, is used. Any resemblance of initials used to a real persons' initials should be considered a coincidental rather than deliberate. Before getting started, it is important also that we all agree that the human body is the same worldwide, specifically, the color of the skin may be deferent, heights and weights may differ, but the structure and function of human organs is the same worldwide except when there is a congenital or acquired malformation. Consequently, when humans with different skin colors and from different parts of the world are subjected to the same condition; locked up in the same room with plasmodium parasite infested mosquitos, for instance, they will all develop malaria with time. What may differ due to uniqueness of individual genes is severity of malaria. If the same people ate ninety percent carbohydrate diet, drank alcohol indiscriminately, drank sugary drinks regularly, ate little or no vegetables, fruits, and nuts, and ate fatty meat most of the days and live sedentary life without any type of physical activities, each will develop one or more of the following health conditions: Type two diabetes, high blood pressure, high cholesterol, arthritis, and cancer to mention the most common. Contrary to unscientific beliefs of Nigerians, there is no white man and Black man disease. Some diseases may be more commonly seen in one race or geographical area than the other, but never completely absent in any of the races.

Case Number One

GN is a 75-year-old woman with osteoarthritis for a very long time on her ankles, knees, hips, shoulders, and finger joints. She was brought by bicycle to the health and wellness center by her granddaughter. She had a walking stick in her right hand and supported on the left side by her granddaughter. She could barely walk. She stated that she recalled precisely when her ailment started. She claimed that no sooner did her husband die than her brother in-law laid claim of her husband's land she had been cultivating for many years. While the dispute was going on, the village chief allowed her to plant her cassava there since everyone knew her husband was cultivating it before his death. She stated that it was after she returned from harvesting cassava from the farm that her joints' pain began and continued to get worst each year. She has been in constant pain, has difficulty getting out of bed in the morning and out of chairs when she sits down. She has been to three different herbalists and prays regularly and nothing seem to help. She is almost bed ridden. She does not attend church or village meetings anymore unless there is a bicycle and someone willing to take her.

Remarkably, given her age, she had no other complaints, her blood pressure, pulse, and respiration were all normal. She has a good appetite and eats well. She was within her normal weight-range, no constipation and all other symptoms were absent. When I told her, she had osteoarthritis and explained to her that it results from wear and tear of the joints over the years. She did not believe me and argued insistently that it was juju put on the farm by her brother in-law. Reluctantly, she accepted high dose strength of ibuprofen on trial basis. After three days, she was brought back, but walked freely without a walking stick. Now she believed in osteoarthritis and not juju as the cause of her pains. She was counseled to walk every day in addition to taking ibuprofen with food and a full cup of water. Osteoarthritis gets worst with sedentary lifestyle, moving the joints by walking and doing the balancing, flexibility and stretch exercises we discussed earlier are approved non-medical treatments for osteoarthritis.

There are three main reasons patients with osteoarthritis do not get lasting relief from pain; the pain drugs in the market are substandard, patients take under dose and do not take it as directed by the prescriber. Osteoarthritis is a chronic illness that is not cured but manageable to provide a client enough relief to be able to perform activities of daily living. Pain drugs are to be taken when there is pain and stop when pain lessens or resolved.

Case Number Two:

NC is a 46-year-old woman who has been married for four years. She claimed to have been pregnant for the last two years and has not been able to deliver because her mother in-law has used voo-doo on her. To the best of her recollection, she had early symptoms of pregnancy such as early morning nausea, vomiting and abdominal movements to suggest fetal presence. Her abdomen is enlarged like eight months pregnancy. On palpation of her abdomen, it was solid like a rock and fibroid was suspected. Ultrasound (scan) imaging confirmed the presence of multiple fairly large fibroids filling her uterus. Fibroid (**oke eghe**) is abnormal growth of smooth muscles of the womb **(figure 18).**

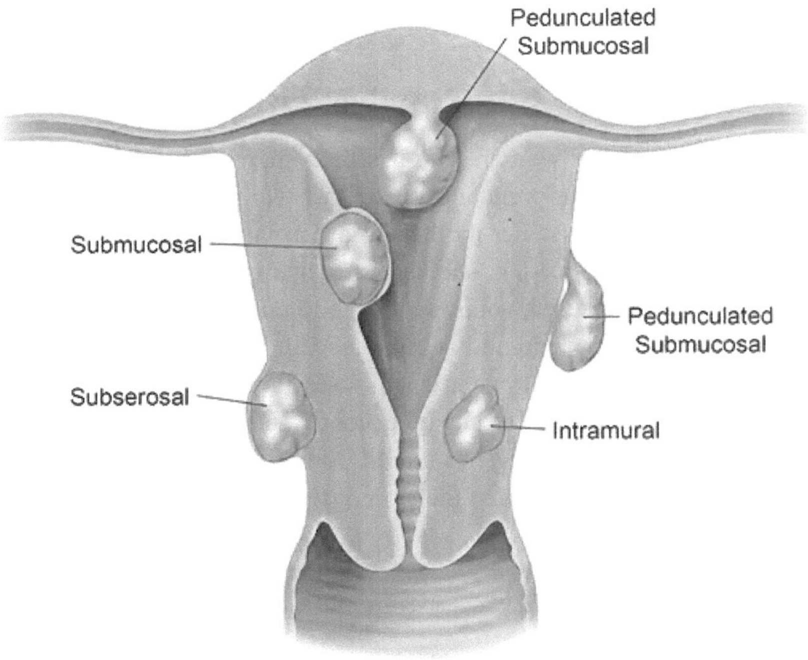

Figure 18

She had surgery that removed her entire womb (total hysterectomy) but left the two ovaries intact. She reluctantly agreed to hysterectomy and had many questions about the after effect. She believed hysterectomy will make her less a woman and affect her sexuality. This false belief is also very common among women in Nigeria. However, the only role of the womb is to house the fetus for nurturing till delivery. After a woman has had all her children, the womb becomes a liability that can develop cancer. In some developed countries, women request total removal of their uterus at the birth of their last child. The ovaries and the adrenal glands on top of each kidneys are responsible for producing hormones which maintain womanhood appearance. Hysterectomy without removing the ovaries does not affect libido and other sexual functions in a woman. NC came to believe that she had been wrong about her mother in-law, whom she has not been in speaking terms for many years. She voluntarily apologized to her and normalized their relationship. Then, she became an evangelist of fibroid awareness, preaching to her friends about what happened to her and how their beliefs in use of juju to prevent conception is all wrong. Fibroid is a common benign growth in the womb (uterus). It can be one or many and does not prevent a woman from conceiving. However, depending on its location and size, it can prevent implantation of a fertilized egg or cause implanted fetus to abort. It is not cancerous but can coexist with cancer of uterus. Fibroids can also coexist with pregnancy without interrupting the pregnancy until normal birth.

It is advisable for woman to have their children as soon as possible, as every woman is at risk for fibroid. In medical books, it is said that any womb that is denied pregnancy consoles itself with fibroid. The older a woman gets, her chance of developing fibroid increases. Although science has not yet uncovered definitively all the things responsible for inducing its development, genetics and hormones are two known culprits. Fibroids run in a family, and it is important that everyone know their family medical history. If your mother, sister, or aunt has had fibroids, you are at higher risk for it than someone without family history, but you may never develop it. I have attended to women who told me that the laboratory scientist drew their blood, did test, and reported that they have fibroid. There is no laboratory blood test to determine if you have fibroids. Ultrasound (Scan) is an imaging test that gives objective confirmation of fibroid presence in the uterus. Ultrasound is more readily available and has no side effects because it does not use radiation. Computed tomography scan (CT-Scan) and Magnetic resonance imaging (MRI) can detect fibroids but are not routinely used because they involve use of radiation that can cause cancer. A good doctor, especially specialists of obstetrics and gynecology can identify fibroid by palpation during physical examination. Still, ultrasound is required to confirm its presence. There are no known drugs, vitamins, or herbs proven yet to shrink or dissolve fibroid. The definitive treatment for fibroid is surgery. And fibroids are treated only if they are causing symptoms like pain, abnormal bleeding, or found to be responsible for infertility. In women approaching menopause with confirmed fibroid that is not causing any problems, no treatment is required. Because fibroid feeds on hormones to grow and persist, after menopause the ovaries involute and do not produce hormones anymore leading to fibroid shrinkage.

Case Number Three:

TS is a 37-year-old woman married for three years. She came in complaining of nausea, vomiting, missed period for about three months and increased appetite. On examination, her abdomen was swollen but the uterus was empty on palpation, and on listening to the abdomen, no fetal heartbeat was detected. The ultrasound result showed an enlarged womb without any fetus in it. TS has false pregnancy also known as pseudopregnancy and clinically as pseudocyesis. Pseudopregnancy is not an uncommon phenomenon and occurs in women who believe they are expecting a child when they are not really carrying a baby. It is seen in women who are suffering from infertility and are desperate, had miscarriage previously, in menopause or desiring to get married. These women experience many if not all symptoms of pregnancy; missed menstruation, nausea, vomiting, swollen belly, enlarged breasts, weight gain and even sensation of fetal movement. It is not known exactly how it occurs, but it is believed that intense desire to become pregnant can cause the body to "believe" that it is pregnant. The brain then misinterprets these psycho-emotional persistent feeling, induce body signals that cause production of pregnancy-hormones: estrogen, progesterone, and prolactin to be released. These hormones lead to the production of true pregnancy symptoms. Risk factors thought to predispose to pseudopregnancy are poverty, lack of education, childhood sexual abuse or relationship problems. I am going to add cultural false beliefs, as it is the case in Nigeria culture. In Nigeria, no sooner does a lady get married than all eyes, especially those of mother in-laws and sister in-laws focus on her abdomen for pregnancy. The newly wed understands she is under intense watch to get pregnant, a "toxic" cultural expectation. She then experiences intense psychological pressure and stress. As pregnancy does not happen quickly, and time continues to fly, the psychological pressure intensifies and trick the body to "thinking" it is pregnant. Also, this intense stress does disrupt the critical normal level and balance of pregnancy-hormones so essential to conceiving and sustaining pregnancy, creating a vicious cycle that delays conception further.

Let's discuss one case of this type. False pregnancy is different from a woman claiming to be pregnant for financial benefits. I have dealt with some such cases whereby sisters, sisters-in-law and friends have called relatives abroad claiming to be pregnant requesting financial assistance. After they receive the money, months later they claim to have lost the pregnancy. I had a case where a sister in-law claimed she was going for delivery and was sent one hundred and fifty thousand naira. And she called weeks later stating she had a dead fetus. But thorough investigation later confirmed she was never pregnant. False pregnancy is also different from delusional pregnancy whereby a schizophrenia (crazy) woman will be broadcasting that she is pregnant when she is not but has a swollen abdomen. Although she is schizophrenic and has the delusion of being pregnant, this can eventually lead to her developing a false pregnancy.

Case Number Four:

CN is a 40-year-old woman who has been married for four years. She presents with a claim of being pregnant for two years and a month. She could not get pregnant in the first two years of her marriage, and the husband and her were led to a woman who gave them some herbs and other drugs. They followed her instructions in bed. After about a month or so, she went for a follow up and she tested her with a computer machine (unspecified), not ultrasound, and pronounced that she was pregnant. She was told she has cryptic pregnancy which can be in the uterus or outside the uterus, and is not detectable by any laboratory or imaging medical testing and could last for several years. Her reason for consulting me is to help her deliver the baby for less cost as she and her husband could not raise the one million, two hundred thousand naira the lady was demanding to deliver the baby.

When assessed, she honestly said she did not know what symptoms of pregnancy feels like since she has never been pregnant before. She said she has never missed her menstruation; it has always been regular lasting three to four days each time. She did not feel nausea, vomiting, increased, or decreased appetite, no weight gain, no swollen abdomen, and no engorgement of the breasts since the two years she was told she is pregnant. These are symptoms of pregnancy of which none has been present. Her physical examination revealed no swollen abdomen and no other signs of pregnancy. An ultrasound test before delivery induction could be done was recommended since she is not in labor. This will show the objective evidence of presence of a child in her womb. She agreed and ultrasound revealed no fetus in the womb or anywhere else in the abdomen. However, there were two small fibroids, one inside and the other outside on top of the womb.

Cryptic or stealth pregnancy is one in which a woman is pregnant and does not know it until one day she goes into labor and has a child. For reasons still elusive to science, symptoms of pregnancy do not appear, as such, these women have no need to do any tests for pregnancy. Women with cryptic pregnancy will not have monthly menstruation but may be bleeding or spotting which they may confuse as menstruation. In fact, the reason cryptic pregnancy is less common is that most women seek health care when their menstruation stops or irregular. It is during this medical visit that tests show that in absence of all early pregnancy symptoms that she is pregnant. These women would not have known that they were pregnant if not for the abnormal bleeding that prompted them to visit a doctor. Lack of pregnancy symptoms results in these women not seeking for pregnancy testing and these are what CN's care giver has manipulated to give her a cooked-up explanation of cryptic pregnancy as a pregnancy that does not show up in any medical test, can implant inside or outside the womb and may last for several years. Menstruation involves sloughing off the inner surface of the womb, stripping all the small blood vessels and thickened tissues that was prepared in anticipation of fetal implant that never happened. Therefore, if a woman is pregnant and was to menstruate at the same time, the fetus will be eliminated with the menstrual material.

Ectopic pregnancy is when the fetus implants outside the uterus. Abdominal pregnancy is a type of ectopic pregnancy, and it is very rare. Abdominal pregnancy is estimated to occur in a ratio of one in ten thousand (1:10,000) pregnancies. When abdominal pregnancy occurs, it will be identified by ultrasound but may be missed in some cases since it is located outside the uterus. In fact, abdominal and pelvic ultrasounds are ordered separately in medicine. When a doctor orders a pelvic ultrasound in a woman having abnormal vaginal bleeding, the sonographer will not on their own do abdominal ultrasound as well. If such a patient has abdominal ectopic pregnancy, it will be missed since abdominal ultrasound was not ordered and was never done. This is contrary to what the care giver to CN has told her that no ultrasound or any other medical test can identify a child outside the womb. Abdominal pregnancies usually cause massive bleeding and are promptly removed surgically as medical emergency. Clues to abdominal pregnancy is when a pregnant woman began to have abdominal pain, pain that is severe when the baby is moving, when the baby is easy to feel or seen easily with ultrasound.

Usually if a doctor discovers abdominal pregnancy early, it is removed by surgery. For the ones that reach second or third trimester, they are delivered by surgery and the placenta is left to be reabsorbed over time. However, there will be ongoing monitoring of the placenta with ultrasound to ensure its complete disappearance. An attempt to surgically remove the placenta will result in massive bleeding that may compromise the life of the mother.

Case Number Five:

ZN is a 30-year-old woman who has been unable to conceive for four years of her marriage. She stated her husband, a primary school classmate, and her have remained together ever since. She reported that she slept only with her husband. Her assessment and physical examination were all normal. She had no other medical problems. Her period was regular and normal in days of flow. However, she was very anxious and stressed and appeared anemic and underweight. Her laboratory test result confirmed she was anemic and five pounds below her normal healthy weight range. Her husband was assessed and sent for laboratory testing. He also was anemic, normal weight and sperm count.

ZN and her husband were given appropriate treatment for anemia, and ZN received additional vitamins to help balance her hormones and one-on-one counseling for stress and anxiety reduction. When a woman has no reproductive system abnormality that could cause infertility, her husband has normal sperm count and they are having intercourse at the critical time range for conception, the most common cause of lack of conception is stress that destabilizes the woman's hormones. Within three months of ZN first consultation, she conceived and had a baby girl nine months later.

Infertility is absence of conception by a couple who have had intercourse at the appropriate time each month for one year. A woman's ovum (egg) lives for 12 to 24 hours. Sperm lives about five days inside a woman. There are six days a woman can get pregnant during each monthly cycle: five days leading to ovulation and twenty-four hours after ovulation. Intercourse within these six critical days ensures conception may take place. Intercourse outside these six days is just for pleasure. It takes one sperm to get pregnant, but on the average, when a man releases sperms it is about 100 million per milliliter.

It is believed that so many sperms are needed since the journey from the cervix to the last one-third part of the fallopian tube where most fertilization take place is a very long journey that few sperms can survive. Nature, therefore, makes available enough sperms to compete so that the healthiest will make it first. A man is considered to have low sperm count if he has less than 15 million per milliliter or 39 million sperms per ejaculation. Contrary to popular believe that when a couple is unable to conceive, it is always a problem from the woman, the problem could be from the man, the woman or both. There are many things that can cause infertility in the man as well as the woman. Both man and woman must be evaluated when they are unable to achieve conception. Couples get better results and quickly do so if they identify an experienced doctor and consistently follow the recommendations of the doctor. Most couples waste irreplaceable valuable time by running from one native doctor, prayer warrior and regular doctor to the other following the directions of their friends and family members. In addition, this run around shopping creates intense anxiety and pressure due to preoccupation with imagination of what people might be saying. Treatment of infertility requires patience, compliance, consistency, and money.

Case Number Six:

MU is a 39-year-old man, who has type two diabetes, hypertension, and high cholesterol for six years. He is married with two children. He is a primary school teacher with National certificate in education. He takes three drugs: glucophage, amlodipine and atorvastatin respectively for his three illnesses. He stated that he takes them religiously. However, he has been unable to bring down his sugar, blood pressure and cholesterol. On assessing him, it became obvious he was not eating properly with respect to his illnesses, was not exercising and was under stress. His laboratory tests showed his sugar to be 372mg/dl,(normal below 100mg/dl) total cholesterol was 293mg/dl (normal below 200mg/dl) and blood pressure was 181/102 mmHg (normal below 120/80mmHg). MU was a walking time bomb. MU was given drugs of the same names from America (glucophage, amlodipine and atorvastatin) he has been buying in Nigeria for all the three illnesses. He also received thirty minutes of intense health education with focus on his current three illnesses. Emphasis was on diet, exercise, stress reduction and strict compliance with taking his drugs as directed. His wife was with him and took note of diet recommendations. He was told to eat and drink, exercise, and reduce stress as described in previous chapters. After one week, his sugar, blood pressure and cholesterol came down significantly but not to the normal range. Within three months, all his test results became normal.

There are many things that either separately or collectively were responsible for MU's previous abnormal test results. First MU was eating and drinking as he wished without considering his health conditions. He was a ticking time-bomb for stroke, and/or heart attack with each having potential to lead to premature death. I consider diabetes, hypertension, and high cholesterol as "three axis of evil for premature death." Medically, they are considered silent killers. MU, or anyone else who has one, two or all three illnesses must reduce consumption of sugar, all carbohydrates and products made from flour. In place of all these, MU must eat all types of beans, vegetables, and nuts. MU must cook with olive oil, vegetable oil, groundnut oil, but not palm oil. Palm oil must be used in a very minute quantity. All oils must be used in moderation. His regular drink must be water with some of it as alkaline water. MU must get at least thirty minutes of exercise every day that includes combination of all four exercise types discussed previously. MU must utilize some of the stress reduction techniques described previously. MU's tests could have remained abnormal despite his religiously taken his Nigerian-market drugs, because the drugs were substandard. It is an undisputed fact that most drugs in Nigerian markets are ineffective because, though their names are right, they contain little or no active ingredients meant to effect healing. Another possibility that is very common in Nigeria is non-compliance with instructions on how to take the drugs. However, MU insisted on being compliant and this was ruled out as contributory to his abnormal laboratory results.

A very common practice of people who have either one or all these three axis-of-evil illnesses, and other chronic but medically manageable illnesses, is the tendency to stop taking drugs when blood pressure, blood sugar and/or cholesterol level drop to normal range. This is a dangerous mistake; test results are normal because of the therapeutic level of drug in the blood stream. Drugs do not stay in the body forever. The body breaks them down and remove the inactive biproducts from the body through urine, sweat and breath. When the critical therapeutic level of blood pressure drug that keeps it down drops because you stopped taking your drugs after your last blood pressure reading shows it normal, you have set yourself up for stroke, heart attack or death. With the blood therapeutic level of the drug low, blood pressure shoots up rapidly. The same is true for blood sugar and cholesterol levels. You must understand and believe that these three illnesses are known as "silent killers" that may show no symptoms or signs while the damage they cause continues to take effect until sudden stroke, heart attack or death. This is not caused by witches, wizards or evil spirits invoked and sent by someone. The knowledge of how all these sudden death happen are well studied, documented and available in public domain.

Case Number Seven:

FE is a 65-year-old man seen on a routine wellness screening during medical mission outreach. He is slim built with no medical complaints. He said he has been in good health for as long as he remembers himself. He described his eating habit as follows: fufu (swallow) daily, about six slices of bread with sugar and milk every morning, drinks alcohol (as much as available) daily, drinks sugary drinks when available, drinks less than three cups of water daily, eats small vegetables, and seldom eats fruits and nuts. He denied smoking or snuffing and does no formal exercise except what he gets moving around as a carpenter. His blood pressure was taken by a nurse twice and it averaged 201/110mmHg (normal is less than 120/80mmHg). He was asked to rest for about twenty minutes and a doctor recorded 195/102mmHg. He denied ever having headaches or any other symptoms related to such high blood pressure. He was given anti-hypertensive drugs immediately and asked to rest. He took home a six-month supply of anti-hypertensive drug, and was educated on lifestyle modification about diet, exercise and stress management then asked to follow up with a primary doctor for thorough physical examination and laboratory tests.

FE was a time-bomb and could have had a heart attack and/or stroke at any moment. His level of blood pressure is silently damaging the eye, kidneys, heart, and brain because these four organs are most vulnerable due to the tiny blood vessels that supply their cells. These tiny blood vessels have very thin walls that can rupture easily under high pressure and lead to blindness, kidney failure, heart attack or stroke. This case underscores the need for at least once a year a doctor's visit for a complete physical examination. FE must change his eating habits, increase exercise, and reduce stress as discussed previously.

Case Number Eight

NN is a 42-year-old woman seen routinely during medical mission screening. She has been married for 10 years with three children. About three years ago, she noticed a small pimple-sized rash surrounded by reddish discoloration near her right breast nipple. However, it was not painful, but would itch every now and then. An ultrasound showed the rash to have extension inside. She was referred for further evaluation during which it was confirmed by biopsy as breast cancer. NN was presented with various treatment options, but she chose to pray. Several attempts to reach her for follow up failed, but three years later she called. She honestly admitted having been praying and taking herbs from native doctors. Now she is ten pounds underweight, has no appetite, a swollen arm that extends into the armpit and excruciating pain. She was confirmed to have metastatic stage four breast cancer. She began chemotherapy and radiotherapy immediately however she tolerated these treatments for about seven months before she succumbed to cancer. When it comes to any illness, delay is very dangerous, especially for cancer. NN demonstrated two things most Nigerians do when they became sick: delay seeking for care and seeking for care in the wrong places.

As stated earlier, every illness has a widow of opportunity within which treatment is most effective and cure can be achieved. Delay misses this widow and cure becomes impossible. And this is most important for all cancer types because cancer cells that refused to die are persistently growing and spreading, destroying normal cells by overcrowding and depriving them of nutrients. The three conventional treatments for breast and other cancers are surgery, chemotherapy, and radiotherapy. It is only in rare but small cases that these three treatment modalities cure cancer. Chemotherapy and radiotherapy destroy both normal and cancer cells. Neither of the two can distinguish normal from cancer cells, hence they have severe side effects. Only immune system cells can distinguish normal from cancer cells. Consequently, methods to boost, speed up and optimize the immune cells' actions are the focus of current cancer treatment research. Meanwhile natural medicine has long shown that high dose Vitamin C works synergistically with some amino acids, minerals and phytonutrient extract of green tea and other herbs to kill cancer cells directly as well as prevent cancer spreading.

For all cancers, early identification and treatment is the key to cure. Women are advised to check their breasts once every month. This is known as self-breast examination (SBE). When you see something on the breast that was not there the month before, you immediately report it to a doctor. Do not be afraid or if you become afraid, overcome it as soon as possible and see a doctor. Delay is very dangerous, especially with cancer. Cancer cells are "intelligent" and will go to any length to deprive normal cells nutrients. Not all things on the breast are cancer. Only doctors are adequately trained to tell breast cancer apart from other diseases of the breast. Pictures and videos that demonstrate how to do self-breast examination can be found on the internet and YouTube. Clinical breast examination should be part of the annual physical examination done by a woman's personal doctor.

A premier requirement for healing any illness is acceptance of the reality of the illness. It is when a sick person assumes the sick role and believe that a problem does exist that he or she would seek for solution to it. But, in many cases for many Nigerians, when there is a health challenge, they recoil into denial mode by saying loudly "I reject it." Friends, family members and church pastor will reinforce the denial by encouraging with "brother or sister reject it, it is not your portion." Even as the individual gets worst daily, he is encouraged to reject it and pray. Another deceitful axiom is " I do not claim it." Church members, family, and friends echo "sister or brother, do not claim it." Either the sick claims it and do something about it timely, or it will claim the sick. Does prayer work? Yes. But it does not often work alone. A sick person must pray as many times as he or she wishes and even enlist other people to pray on their behalf. However, he must also seek out treatments from trained health providers for their illness. Didn't the Bible teach that faith without work is dead in itself?

Case Number Nine:

MN is a 74-year-old retired banker with known hypertension, high cholesterol, low back pain and arthritis on multiple joints but more severe on the right knee. He stated that he takes his drugs regularly which are usually sent from London by his daughter who is a nurse and husband is a doctor. One morning he had an urge to urinate, and he quickly ran into the bathroom but could not urinate. He was in such discomfort he had never experienced before in his entire life. He was rushed to the hospital where a catheter was inserted to let urine out. He was diagnosed with an enlarged prostate that closed off the urinary tract (urethra) through which urine runs out from the bladder. Enlarged prostate also known as benign prostate hypertrophy is very common among men worldwide and every man is at risk. MN did admit that for about a year or so, he must push hard to urinate and takes long to finish as the streaming runs very slowly. He was discharged with appropriate drugs that will help shrink the prostate and keep the urethra open.

The urethra in man runs through the center of the prostate as it leaves the bladder. The prostate is normally the size of a walnut, but as men get older, it gets bigger. Gene and male hormone; testosterone, is suspected to play role in the enlargement of prostate, but other unidentified factors may be involved. Surgery is only used as a last resort in complete urethral closure like the case of MN if appropriate drugs taken correctly is not helpful. Pumpkin seed contains phytochemicals that has been shown to shrink the prostate. Benign prostate hypertrophy is a chronic illness for which drugs must be taken for life. When drugs are stopped, with time the urethra will close completely once again, and surgery becomes necessary.

Note that both MN and his doctor exhibited negligence towards his prostate. It seems that MN never acquainted his doctor with his urination difficulties over the years. And it seems that his doctor did not ask about his prostate during history and physical examination. It is common for both doctor and patient to focus on obvious symptoms and signs of presently presenting illnesses, in the case of MN, hypertension, high cholesterol and arthritis without complete review of the body systems. It is your responsibility as a patient to tell your doctor everything. Ignoring discussions that involve sexual organs is a cultural pitiful that must be relinquished during healthcare visits. Problems of penis, vagina and breasts do kill just like diabetes and hypertension. Breast cancer is the most common cancer death in women in all cultures. Yet breast cancer is a curable cancer diseases if identified early by a woman who is diligent in monthly self-breast examination and seeks medical care for any observed change as soon as seen. You do not have to wait till your doctor asks. If your doctor is of the opposite gender, there should be no shame, he/she has seen it all through medical school and practice.

Case Number Ten:

GN is a 39-year-old man on admission in a Nigerian hospital for 10 days. GN's sister called and reported he woke up one morning paralyzed, unable to move his hands and legs but could speak softly. On direct assessment, GN stated that he had sore throat, fever, and tiredness unrelated to physical work two weeks ago. He further said that a few days before his body shot down, he had tingling and numbness on his toes. His sister was very distraught, complained that for ten days in the hospital, nothing else had been done except tests and more tests. All the while, her brother began having a problem breathing and the hospital staff were not telling her and the rest of the family what was going on. The patient was transferred to another hospital in another city by my recommendation and was discharged after one month of stay. He recovered fully on outpatient in about nine months without complications or disability. However, there were several theories floating in the village about what happened to him, such as: because he refused to get married (he is the last born) his deceased father bewitched him, and spirit attack invoked by one of his age-group meeting member he had quarreled with about eight days preceding his illness.

These erroneous theories rooted in health illiteracy and superstition were reinforced by the failure of the first hospitals not being able to name his illness. In fact, the sister said she was advised by a nurse in the hospital when the hospital decided to discharge him to seek native doctor solution. GN had an illness known as Guillain-Barre Syndrome (GBS), a rare autoimmune disorder in which the immune system attacks and destroys the coat of nerves known as myelin. The cause is not known but it usually follows viral infection of respiratory or gastro-intestine system.

For this reason, it is speculated that this is a case of mistaken identity whereby the nervous system is an innocent bystander that shares a surface protein with a virus that infects the respiratory or gastro-intestine tract. The immune cells therefore mistake the nerves as the invading parasite and destroy the myelin sheath insulating the nerves. Usually, the sheath coating of nerves known as myelin insulates the nerves and ensure propagation of nerve impulse to and from the brain. With myelin destroyed, impulses do not reach the brain hence general body paralysis. GBS is more common in men, especially young men than women. There is no known cure for GBS, however, most patients recover fully within a year.

There are many illnesses like GBS, and their unusual nature tend to reinforce the superstitious beliefs in witches and wizards as their cause. In medicine, it is said that if a doctor does not think about an illness, he may never diagnose it. Expressed in a more common way; you cannot find what you are not looking for. It is alarming to hear from family members how often hospitals discharge their loved ones to go and try native doctors.

Case Number Eleven:

EE is 47 years old man who walked into Health and Wellness Center office about 5 pm and slummed onto a couch complaining of tiredness not attributable to physical exhaustion. He has been a construction company administration executive for 11 years and sits in the office for most of his work. He denied any prior medical problems, his father died at age 61 from heart attack and mother died at age 73 from stroke after suffering from high blood pressure and high cholesterol diagnosed four months preceding her death. He has two brothers and a sister who have no known medical problems. He further complained of frequent severe headaches that responds mildly to Ibuprofen. He sleeps less than five hours a night. He has never smoked but says he drinks socially.

However, on probing further, he admits drinking every day after work with some co-workers and sometimes gets back home very late. He could not remember the exact age at which he began drinking but could only say he began drinking very young. He volunteered that his wife has voiced concerns about his drinking and suggested for him to reduce or stop all together. His sex life is in the pits, meaning he does not achieve nor sustain erection. He could not recall the last time he visited a doctor and had never had any annual physical examination.

His blood pressure was 160/101 mmHg and pulse 96. He was oozing strong alcohol breath and sweating profusely despite that the sun has gone down.

Examination of his heart with electrocardiography machine suggests that his heart was enlarged. Ultrasound confirmed enlarged and failing heart and liver. Laboratory examination of his blood shows that he had elevated cholesterol and enzymes indicating that he has been drinking more and longer than he admitted.

Putting all these together shows that EE has an alcohol drinking problem, which earns him diagnosis of alcoholic. I comfortably can add alcoholism to the growing list of diseases known as silent killers. As it is obvious from the tests conducted on him, EE has failing heart and liver which accounts for his exhaustion, fatigue, and tiredness due to heavy protracted alcohol consumption. Alcohol misuse and abuse has adverse consequences, of which some are immediate during intoxication, and others during withdrawal stage. However, it damages the internal organs slowly and silently without obvious symptoms and signs until permanent damage occurs. As stated earlier, alcohol is a drug unlike any other drug known to damage every part of human body when used in large quantity for long time. Detailed specific damage and illnesses related to disease of alcohol is the subject of future booklet.

The cornerstone of alcohol treatment is total and complete abstinence. There has been debates about whether an alcoholic can learn to drink responsibly and socially. So far, the evidence clearly shows that it is almost impossible. The natural course of disease of alcoholism is that of relapse and remission. The natural tendency for an alcoholic in remission for several months or years is to spiral down to full relapse once he picks the first drink. Although there are available prescription drugs for helping cut the craving, as well as ones to help avert picking the drink up in the first place, their success is very limited due to the inherent nature of the intense overwhelming craving and desire to drink when the right cues are present. To strive and achieve complete abstinence is the only means to avoid premature death from disease of alcoholism. One good news is that complete recovery of major body organs is possible if an alcoholic stops completely before permanent damage occurs.

Case Number Eleven:

EE is 47 years old man who walked into Health and Wellness Center office about 5 pm and slummed onto a couch complaining of tiredness not attributable to physical exhaustion. He has been a construction company administration executive for 11 years and sits in the office for most of his work. He denied any prior medical problems, his father died at age 61 from heart attack and mother died at age 73 from stroke after suffering from high blood pressure and high cholesterol diagnosed four months preceding her death. He has two brothers and a sister who have no known medical problems. He further complained of frequent severe headaches that responds mildly to Ibuprofen. He sleeps less than five hours a night. He has never smoked but says he drinks socially.

However, on probing further, he admits drinking every day after work with some co-workers and sometimes gets back home very late. He could not remember the exact age at which he began drinking but could only say he began drinking very young. He volunteered that his wife has voiced concerns about his drinking and suggested for him to reduce or stop all together. His sex life is in the pits, meaning he does not achieve nor sustain erection. He could not recall the last time he visited a doctor and had never had any annual physical examination.

His blood pressure was 160/101 mmHg and pulse 96. He was oozing strong alcohol breath and sweating profusely despite that the sun having gone down.

Examination of his heart with electrocardiography machine suggests that his heart was enlarged. Ultrasound confirmed enlarged and failing heart and liver. Laboratory examination of his blood shows that he had elevated cholesterol and enzymes indicating that he has been drinking more and longer than he admitted.

Putting all these together shows that EE has an alcohol drinking problem, which earns him diagnosis of alcoholic. I comfortably can add alcoholism to the growing list of diseases known as silent killers. As it is obvious from the tests conducted on him, EE has failing heart and liver which accounts for his exhaustion, fatigue, and tiredness due to heavy protracted alcohol consumption. Alcohol misuse and abuse has adverse consequences, of which some are immediate during intoxication, and others during withdrawal stage. However, it damages the internal organs slowly and silently without obvious symptoms and signs until permanent damage occurs. As stated earlier, alcohol is a drug unlike any other drug known to damage every part of human body when used in large quantity for long time. Detailed specific damage and illnesses related to disease of alcohol is the subject of future booklet.

The cornerstone of alcohol treatment is total and complete abstinence. There has been debates about whether an alcoholic can learn to drink responsibly and socially. So far, the evidence clearly shows that it is almost impossible. The natural course of disease of alcoholism is that of relapse and remission. The natural tendency for an alcoholic in remission for several months or years is to spiral down to full relapse once he picks the first drink. Although there are available prescription drugs for helping cut the craving, as well as ones to help avert picking the drink up in the first place, their success is very limited due to the inherent nature of the intense overwhelming craving and desire to drink when the right cues are present. To strive and achieve complete abstinence is the only means to avoid premature death from disease of alcoholism. One good news is that complete recovery of major body organs is possible if an alcoholic stops completely before permanent damage occurs.

Case Number Twelve:

KO is a 79-year-old great grandmother and a retired secondary school teacher. She has had high blood pressure, high cholesterol, arthritis, and cataract for some years. About a year ago, according to her daughter, she began to forget things and will stop in the middle of sentences whether she is speaking English, Igbo, or pidgin English. Recently she could not recognize people she had known for decades including some of her family members. She is not allowed to go out by herself because on several occasions she had gone out and could not find her way back and would be brought back home by outsiders. KO is frustrated most of the time and has been violent unprovoked towards her nurse and house cleaner. KO has a visiting home nurse that ensures she takes drugs regularly and on time. She has a housemaid since she is not able to do her activities of daily living on her own.

KO was confirmed to have Alzheimer's disease; a type of dementia resulting in memory loss. Alzheimer's disease usually affects people 65 years and above, however, some people have a type known as early onset that begin in the 40s and 50s. There is no definitive known external cause for AD, however, having APOE gene predisposes to developing it, while mutation on any of these three other genes; APP, PSEN 1 and PSEN 2 specifically predispose to early onset type of Alzheimer's disease. Some researchers have suggested that AD is diabetes type three because they found evidence that excess sugar is an external trigger to developing the disease. High blood pressure, high cholesterol and sedentary lifestyle are equally suspected culprits to cause Alzheimer's disease. Forgetfulness, confusion, misplacement of objects and inability to perform activities one was used to doing are early warning signs of AD. Currently, there is no cure, but prescription drugs are available thought to be able to slow the progression.

Lifestyle modification with respect to diet, exercise and stress as previously discussed is helpful both for slowing progression, preventing, and delaying onset in a genetically predisposed individual. Like all illnesses, when a family member, especially first-degree relation; a parent, sibling or child has AD, prevention is highly recommended. Oily fish, nuts, Omega-3 (fish oil) and vitamin E supplements are recommended for prevention. AD patients require close observation for wandering away, aggression and self-injury.

Case Number Thirteen:

CA is a 29-year-old married woman with two children. She is an elementary school teacher. She complained of severe pounding headache that only goes away when she takes codeine. At night she does not sleep unless she takes valium. Recently, her friend and co-worker introduced her to using tramadol which she said relieves her headache better than codeine. She said she must take valium several times daily otherwise she will not be able to teach or do anything else. She owes her friends lots of money and a male co-worker gives her money in exchange for sexual favors. She must borrow money to buy these drugs because she must present her entire monthly salary to her husband for household expenses. She is tormented with guilt for not being sure if her husband is truly the father of her two-year-old son. She presented very anxious and depressed.

CA is a classical case that embodies many things wrong with the healthcare system and health illiteracy. She became addicted to codeine inadvertently. She initially had headache and she ran to the chemist, bought codeine which stopped her headache. Next time, she had headache she used codeine to stop the headache. What she did not know is that codeine, valium, and tramadol are all prescription- controlled drugs in developed countries. This means that no one can buy these drugs without a doctor recommending it and they are to be used for a short time. This is because controlled drugs have addictive potential. They may provide immediate calming and pain-relieving effect, but when their effect goes away, there comes a rebound of anxiety, restlessness, more pain, and sweating. These are withdrawal effects due to the absence of the drug in the body system. When the individual takes another dose of the controlled-addictive substance, all the symptoms of withdrawal immediately go away. A vicious cycle is then created that gets the now valium, codeine, or tramadol addict to be running in and out of the drug store.

Worst still, the addict now develop tolerance to the drugs. This means that if 10mg of valium stopped her headache and pain initially, after using 10mg for some time, it becomes ineffective, and she needs 20mg to get same relieving effect. With time she will escalate the dose to a level that will cause death due to overdose. It should be pointed out here that alcohol is a drug that has the same effects as valium, Librium, Codeine, tramadol, the only difference is that it is in liquid form.

CA received intensive counseling overtime and recovered but was clearly informed that the tendency to go back to using must be guarded for her entire life. She was advised to use non-addiction fever, headache and pain drugs like Ibuprofen and Tylenol. CA was a victim of flawed healthcare systems that allows all drugs over-the-count without prescription. However, even in developed countries where the controlled drugs are under prescription and intensely monitored, some patients still get addicted and roam from one doctor to the other with different stories in attempt to obtain their next supply. Drug addiction and alcohol addiction is a public health crisis in Nigeria today.

I must also share that in the early 1990s the first person who came to me with similar case as CA was a woman, an elementary school teacher. She received in-depth cognitive counseling like CA and did very well. However, after about eight months, I was called by a friend of hers to say that she was fatally hit by a car one night when she went to buy something. I later found out that she was hit by a lorry as she was walking out of a drug store about 7 pm. Her daughter confirmed my guess that she was complaining of headache and went to buy drugs. Perhaps I am the only one who know the cause of her death, addiction to valium and codeine. The disease of addiction is perhaps the most complex illness ever. There is no consensus on the question; addiction, is it a moral weakness, a habit, a sin, a curse, a spiritual attack, or disease? The answer depends on whom you ask. I must emphasis that the only cure for disease of addiction is never to start in the first place.

The natural course of all diseases of addiction is relapse and remission roller-coaster that spans the entire life of an individual. While the definitive goal is cure, realistically what is attainable is sustaining remission for as long as possible with diligent mindful guide against relapse. One keyway to achieve this is to identify all the possible cues that triggers relapse and guide against them. Cues are usually people, places, and things universally applicable to all addicts such as a bar for an alcoholic, and other cues that are unique to individual addict such as smell of burning bush for a marijuana addict.

Case Number Fourteen:

SA is a forty-year-old woman, without a child in her current marriage but has three daughters from her previous polygamist marriage. Even before her previous husband died, her and her daughters were treated like outcasts because she had no male child. Things got worst with the sudden death of her husband who provided the only shield she had from the abuse and torment by two older co-wives. In search of a male child, and hopefully escape the torment by her co-wives and their children, she remarried. Although things were going well in her new marriage and she stated that she was comfortable like never before in her life, she felt very sad because she could not get pregnant again. In the first year of her second marriage, she had an ectopic pregnancy that almost cost her life.

SA became suddenly psychotic; hearing voices, and seeing things that were not real, and began to talk to herself. She was initially treated by a native doctor without success. Then she was sent to a church that diagnosed her with harboring demons. The church was to pray and cast out the demons. When I arrived on annual medical mission in 2010, my crew and I went on a Sunday to the church to meet SA . On arrival the congregation was active inside the church building singing loud music. I asked a lady standing in front of the Church building if she knew where SA was. She responded with, "follow me." She took us inside a bush behind that Church building. SA was tied with raffia rope to a tree with multiple wounds all over her and flies hovering around them. We quickly untied her and drove off with her. She was given a bath, fed and her wounds treated. She was at least ten pounds underweight. Within the next three weeks, she responded very well to low dose antipsychotic and anti-depression drugs. She eventually stabilized to her normal self. SA had depression with psychotic features. Her family background did not yield previous case of mental illness. It is my educated belief that SA became depressed due to the treatment she received throughout life, and the now reality that she could not have the male child she desperately craved.

Although her current husband, a widower, had adult children, SA felt she was not useful to the husband since she could not bear him a child. She woke up one day packed her things and went back to her birthplace against all pleading by her husband. SA represent a significant number of people who focus on negative things in their life at complete exclusion of positive things that have happened to them and potential future ones. This is most common among Christian women who have wrongly been indoctrinated by their clergy that if they come to Church regularly, pay their tithes and offerings, they are immune from negative things of life. And when they are challenged by negative things of life, they conclude that God has abandoned them, and depression sets in. The corner stone treatment for this type of depression caused by perceived false beliefs and misinterpretation of situations is a combination of low dose antidepressant and intense extended cognitive psychotherapy (counseling) that explains the truth of situation of things to the individual. These individuals need to adopt in practice the axiom; change your thought to change your life. The culture of must-have a male child to carry the family name has caused devastating blows to many individuals and families. A female child carries the same fifty percent of her father's genes as her brothers. When she marries outside, her children will carry the same quarter gene of her father as well as her brother's children. Many daughters today are not married for various reasons to be discussed elsewhere. Are these daughters to be denied building houses and having children in their father's compound? The new normal happening now that will never go away is that a daughter can have children and build in her father's compound if she is approaching the end of reproductive age and no husband in sight. No one applied to be born and let alone to be born a male or female. Cultures are, and should remain dynamic, and not static.

Based on what I have experienced for more than three decades, and in many countries, and cultures, everyone must strive to have a female child. With only rare exceptions, when old age and/or illness strikes, it is almost always the daughters that are present to provide needed care.

Women in this regard are like two-edged sword. A daughter will go against all the objections of her husband and secretly provide for her parents yet may not allow her parent in-laws to come to their son's house. And your son, if not strong willed, may only care for you to the extent his wife allows. All these may seem to be relational issues, but they have severe mental and physical health consequences.

Case Number Fifteen:

ZI is a 36-year-old man with two children under six years. His wife is CI a 33-year-old woman eight months pregnant. At the nineth month she went into labor and was rushed to a general hospital. At the hospital, she was admitted but left on attended. I was contacted from Nigeria, and I sent a nurse to the hospital. When the nurse arrived, she confirmed that CI was very weak with barely palpable purse. Blood pressure was very low, and the heartbeat of her fetus was not detectable. The hospital staff was not answering questions and there was no other way to determine if she was ever fed while she was left abandoned. As a result of my previous experience with this type of case, my suspicion was confirmed when I asked the nurse to check the contents of CI's handbag. She found bottles of prescription drugs and when she read their names out, they were all drugs for treating human immunodeficiency virus and acquired immune deficiency syndrome (HIV/AIDS).

As late as 2010, HIV positive pregnant women in Nigeria were abandoned in labor to die. And many, I mean many died this way at a time when options where readily available to deliver these women with the medical personal protected with personal protective equipment. CI died as well as her fetus. ZI tested HIV positive and was stunned. Although he looked very healthy and appeared to be about his ideal healthy weight, he would lapse into profound depression. He said he never knew his wife was HIV positive. She was traveling on business trips and would be gone for days, while ZI was working and comes home to stay with the children. Suddenly, ZI became seriously sick and died six months later. Although ZI had a chance to beat HIV as he was relatively in good health and drugs were available and many more was coming out that we hoped and today they are, would make HIV a chronic disease and not necessarily deadly one it was at the beginning. ZI never recovered from the devastation of being betrayed by his wife and died from broken heart and not HIV. He did not even develop AIDS. I had several discussions with him, and he did not come out of his depression. His last words as I was on the phone with him was, "look after the children." Can someone die of a broken heart? Yes. It happens every day.

Summing Up

I have laid out many of the ways humans get sick. Skin colors apart, human structure and function is the same worldwide. However, there are individual uniqueness due to genetic variations which confers, among other things, individual resilience to causes of different sickness. We discussed that illness results from nature mistakes, competition among living things for survival, eating and drinking habits, accidents, sedentary lifestyle, and effects of environmental factors on human body. There is no evidence of existence of witches, wizards and evil spirits that cause any known human sickness. We discussed the role alteration in normal balance of neurotransmitters and hormones play in causing both physical and mental sickness. The concept of evil spirit, witches and wizards is a construct of human mind; beliefs and thoughts that accumulate as a result. For instance, if someone walking down the road during a heavy rain gets struck by a lightning and he dies, he was not killed by an evil spirit, witches, wizards, sin he or his ancestors committed, rather physics has a clear authentic explanation of how currents from the lightening flows through his body which acted as conductor to cause his death. He was at the wrong place at the wrong time.

We discussed various ways to avoid getting sick by being mindful of what we eat, drink, being active and not sedentary and reducing stress through various techniques. Going for at least once a year for a complete physical examination is recommended in order to uncover early stages of various illnesses that do not show any symptoms until it is late. Diabetes, hypertension, and high cholesterol are what I dubbed three axis of evil that seldom elicit overt symptoms but continue to subtly cause damages that suddenly can lead to stroke, heart attack or fatality. For this fact, they are known as silent killers. We discussed the right things you must do when you get sick. Going to see a doctor as soon as possible, taking a companion with you, making list of all the questions you must ask the doctor about your concerns, taking with you all the prescriptions, non-prescriptions drugs, vitamins, minerals, and herbs you are taking, letting the doctor know all other alternative and complementary treatments you are using, making sure that the doctor lists legibly all drugs and recommendations given to you, asking for explanations when not clear, getting full name of the doctor (Dr. John Jackson), not Dr. Jackson as he is not the only Dr. Jackson, obtain phone number to call if any problems, such as when side effect occurs from taking any of the drug the doctor prescribed. It is your life, your only life, you are solely responsible for it not the doctor, nurse, or hospital. It is recommended that you set aside a portion of your daily earnings for emergency health problems. The main reason we get sick is because we are alive. Dead people do not get sick. Being a devote Christian, born again, devote Muslim or any other religious faith does not provide you immunity from sickness. Praying several times daily, reading religious books daily, or paying tithes regularly will not prevent anyone from getting sick occasionally.

The best evidence shows that keeping your immune system functioning at its optimal capacity will prevent most illness, delay most illness, help you recover quickly when you get sick, but does not virtually eliminate the possibility of getting sick. Learning the resources that provide for a strong immune system is the key to living healthily and longer. The truth about healing is that the body heals itself and no drug does. All drugs are only helpers to the immune system in its healing assignment. Even when chemotherapy and radiotherapy succeed in killing cancer cells, the cellular debris left is cleared by the immune cells. If cellular debris is left to accumulate, it will lead to another sickness that may be fatal. For your healthy living and long life, learn and live.

Synopsis

Why and How We Get Sick, Not by Witches and Wizards: Unveiling the Science Behind Illness and Health

In this enlightening and accessible book, delve into the fascinating world of medical science to uncover the true causes of illness and the pathways to health. Moving beyond myths and superstitions, **Why and How We Get Sick** demystifies the complex interactions between our bodies and the environment.

Explore how modern science explains the origins of diseases, from infections and genetic disorders to lifestyle-related conditions. Learn about the body's defense mechanisms, the role of nutrition, and the impact of mental health on physical well-being. This book offers a comprehensive guide to understanding how we can protect and enhance our health through evidence-based practices.

Perfect for anyone curious about the science of health, this book is a must-read for those seeking to empower themselves with knowledge and take control of their well-being.

Made in United States
Troutdale, OR
11/03/2026

56845393R00066